Praise for

The Clarity Cleanse and Dr. Habib Sadeghi

"*Trust deeper.* These two words, the journey to understanding them, and the man who taught them to me have changed my life. Dr. Sadeghi's *The Clarity Cleanse* is essential reading for anyone who has felt lost or broken (in other words, for everyone) and wanted to heal into a kinder, stronger, and braver person. I cannot recommend it highly enough."
—Anne Hathaway, actress

"*The Clarity Cleanse*—this is a GAME CHANGER! If you're ready to stop going around in circles you have found your map. *The Clarity Cleanse* is essential for de-cluttering your emotional and physical body giving you more conscious control of your life and a taste of what it is to really live healthy, happy, and free! Doctor Sadeghi is absolutely incredible."
—Demi Moore, actress

"This brilliant and challenging book is also kind and gentle, like its author, the clear, the intensely practical Habib: Add five drops of lavender oil to your bath. A cup of Epsom salts will also help.

By the time you finish reading this, you will have found a new friend."
—Coleman Barks, *The Essential Rumi*

"Habib Sadeghi offers a new perspective on illness and disease and the pitfalls and obstacles that lay in the path of healing. *The Clarity Cleanse* is a fresh and innovative approach to what we can do to live healthier and happier lives."
—Tim Robbins, actor

"Dr. Sadeghi has helped me understand a path of clarity in my life. He's supported me in bridging the connection between mind and body work. I hope others will find healing in his compassionate teachings."
                                                    —Jessica Chastain, actress

"Dr. Sadeghi's insights provide the courage to overcome your fears and surpass your limits. This book empowers people in a way that proves no one has to be the victim of circumstance."
                                                    —Toby Maguire, actor

"In these times, it's imperative that we become aware that our emotional state has a major impact on our physical health. Yet I'm still witnessing people fall ill and settle for treatment that's purely palliative and not curative, as if their emotions and way of thinking have played no part in their illness. *The Clarity Cleanse* is our collective wake-up call. Dr. Habib Sadeghi makes it clearer than ever that if we wish to live in a state of wellness, it's crucial to address our emotions, our attitudes, and our overall state of being.
                                                    —Elena Brower, author of *Practice You*

"*The Clarity Cleanse* demystifies self-improvement in a way that's exciting and accessible. It's common sense approach walks you closer to more power and progress in your life. Thank you, Dr. Sadeghi, for the bravery it took to tell your personal story, and to allow it to heal countless others. I am so grateful to be learning from it."
                                                    —Annabelle Wallis, actress

"Clarity is the key to living a conscious life, and Dr. Sadeghi understands it better than anyone I know. *The Clarity Cleanse* is a practical path to recognizing how we create our life circumstances and consciously putting that power to work in a profound way."
                                                    —Tony Florence, General Partner, NEA Venture Capital

"Dr. Sadeghi reinvents what it means to reinvent yourself, and It's not just about seeing your life clearly but about finding the courage to move forward. He is the number one living proof that through love and gratitude, humans can co-create daily miracles. I'm eternally grateful to him."
—Penelope Cruz, actress

"My loving and caring friend Dr. Sadeghi makes self-empowerment attainable and easy to understand. It's because of what Dr. Sadeghi has overcome in his life that makes his guidance so relevant. He is a soul doctor who facilitates healing light where others might only see sickened darkness."
—Javier Bardem, actor

"Dr. Sadeghi simply saved my life. His rigorous honesty and compassion coupled with his tremendous skill makes him the most valuable voice in medicine. He is direct in both his vision and guidance. This book will you give you the tools to both simplify and amplify for your life for the better. Much like treatment with the man himself, this program will leave you feeling both healed and loved. Oh, and the best part: it's a cleanse with no yucky shakes!"
—Jenni Konner, director, writer, and producer of *Girls*

"*The Clarity Cleanse* offers a profound path to healing. In it, Dr. Sadeghi clearly shows the false duality of mind and body, that indeed the mind and body are one and our internal worlds are constantly and deeply reflected in our physical body. In a very readable, accessible, and understandable manner he demonstrates how negative emotional energy gets trapped in our physical body and can lead to both psychological and physical breakdown, even debilitating disease. Most importantly, he leads us on a tangible 12-step path to healing through the cultivation of Clarity. From cleansing the body and mind, through recognizing repression and finding meaning in suffering, he helps us empty what has been poisonous to our beings, and replace the now available space with a restored life force. He leads us with a sense of safety and security, optimism and hope, on the journey from illness and disease to thriving and flourishing."

—Alane Daugherty, PhD, professor of kinesiology at California State Polytechnic University, Pomona; co-director of the Mind and Heart Research Lab (at Cal Poly); and research consultant for the Center for Engaged Compassion at the Claremont School of Theology

"*The Clarity Cleanse* is a profound and compassionate journey you can take at your own pace. Dr. Sadeghi has changed my life."

—Jennifer Meyer, designer

"In Native American lore, fear is the first enemy of learning to extend our presence into the world. Clarity is the dispeller of our fear of fear and our shame of shame. Dr. Sadeghi demonstrates this by putting his own story on the line. Clarity is described as the containing action beyond control and constriction that allows us to face the obstacles of development with a better-informed intuition. As both a patient and friend, I have experienced this first-hand."

—Gary David, PhD, *Epistemics: The Art of Learning*

"In my professional life, I achieved heights beyond my expectations, but in comparison my personal life was empty. NO ONE should settle for EMPTY! In *The Clarity Cleanse*, Dr. Sadeghi outlined the steps to lead me to my own miracle of finding purpose, growth, and love."

—Jeanie Buss, owner, Los Angeles Lakers

"Working with Dr. Sadeghi for several years has been one of the most powerful and rewarding experiences that I've ever gifted myself. Now, you can do the same for yourself! *The Clarity Cleanse* is an accessible tool to discover your power that comes from within."

—Daniela Villegas, designer

"Life-changing and life-giving, a clear and beautiful way to heal."

—Yolande Yorke-Edgell, choreographer

"It's rare to find a healer who treats the whole person—mind, body, and spirit. Dr. Sadeghi is such a healer, a master at helping people find the emotional and spiritual causes of disease. *The Clarity Cleanse* explains these causes, and offers a practical, essential guide for healing one's whole being. Dr. Sadeghi's 12 step mind-body-spirit cleanse and maintenance program is powerful medicine for removing the obstacles to health and happiness, and puts people back in control over their lives. If you are looking for a pill to make you better, then this is not your book. But if you want to discover the secrets to healing yourself and living a fulfilling life, then you will love this book."

—Sydney Ross Singer, medical anthropologist
and author of *Dressed To Kill*

"If you are looking to go deeper in your life this book contains the answers you have been looking for. Find how to awaken your mind, heart, and body and soul. Find the self-empowerment you never knew you had!"

—Dan McCarroll, former president of
Warner Bros Records and Capitol Records

"An essential guide to creating calm at the center of life's storms and the ability to make self-affirming choices."

—Colin C. Blaydon, PhD, founding director, Center for Private
Equity and Entrepreneurship, Dartmouth University

"As a personal patient of Dr. Habib Sadeghi's, as well as an advocate for his work, I find it remarkable that he has spent the time and care to communicate the ineffable. A few years ago, I was faced with a tragic curveball that one might feel life just threw at them.

How could I find the strength to navigate it while being there for my health and all of those that count on me?

The Clarity Cleanse is an open tutorial of education and practice to help you to realize your fullest potential by breaking down and building up the areas that lie within you of imbalance, misidentification, and weakness, by traveling through your roots to find the wee child inside of you that needs to be nursed to its next level.

This radically honest dive into how to perform this cleanse to clarity will peel away so many of the layers of this life that you feel keep you from living your most honest, empowered, happy, and healthy life. You deserve that, and I for one can attest to how this incredible multidisciplinary genius, Dr. Habib Sadeghi is FOR you."

—Tracy Anderson, creator of the Tracy Anderson Method, and health & fitness expert

"*The Clarity Cleanse* provides the map to the answers we have wondered could exist. It is the portal to self-power, joy, good health, and peace."   —Kurt Rambis, associate head coach, New York Knicks

"*The Clarity Cleanse* is a sobering look at the approach to the healing we have all wondered if such a thing really existed. It starts with opening your intuitive, your heart and the soul of truth to understand the life you are worthy of."   —Michael Watkins, actor

"Dr. Habib Sadeghi, has written a masterful book discussing the energetic causes of illness; the highest and best approach to addressing one's health challenge while empowering us to trust our own intuition, which I believe connects us directly to our own inner physician. One of the more important lines in his book, 'much of the current medical model is trapped in the concrete world, the world of effects, unaware there's an entire unseen world of energy from which everything we observe is created.' Dr. Sadeghi takes us on a journey of greater understanding and awareness regarding ourselves and the world of which we are a part. In my book, I mentioned that if people want change, they are responsible to make those changes happen. *The Clarity Cleanse* provides us with what we need to attain better health and wellbeing.

—Steven A. Ross, PhD, president of the World Research Foundation and author of *And Nothing Happened... But You Can Make It Happen*

"The Clarity Cleanse is a manual for living. We have within us everything we need to create wellness and this book explains how. it will forever change your relationship with illness and reveal the power of how to use "clarity" to heal disease. The knowledge and wisdom contained in this book is a gift to anyone seeking a deeper understanding of how they are functioning psychologically, spiritually, and physically. *The Clarity Cleanse* offers a profound new perspective on our processes of mind and body, the roots of disease and the steps to healing.

As a patient of Dr. Sadeghi's I have experienced firsthand the power of his enlightened healing. after reading this book you will never experience your patterns of thinking and feeling in same way. This book distills Dr. Sadeghi's revolutionary knowledge into a manual for anyone to become the master of their own wellness. Your relationship with your past, those around you, and most importantly with yourself will never be the same. If you are ready to heal yourself, read this book; if you are ready to love yourself, read this book; if you are ready to cleanse yourself, read this book.

May *The Clarity Cleanse* heal those who read it and be the beginning of a new way to live and love."

—Alexis Denisof, actor

The
Clarity
Cleanse

12 STEPS TO
FINDING RENEWED ENERGY,
SPIRITUAL FULFILLMENT,
AND EMOTIONAL HEALING

Habib Sadeghi, DO, FACEMIP

Foreword by
Gwyneth Paltrow

**goop
press**

**GRAND CENTRAL
PUBLISHING**

NEW YORK   BOSTON

Grand Central Publishing
Hachette Book Group
1290 Avenue of the Americas, New York, NY 10104
grandcentralpublishing.com
twitter.com/grandcentralpub

Originally published in hardcover by Grand Central Life & Style in December 2017
First trade paperback edition: December 2019

Grand Central Publishing is a division of Hachette Book Group, Inc. The Grand Central Publishing name and logo is a trademark of Hachette Book Group, Inc.

The publisher is not responsible for websites (or their content) that are not owned by the publisher.

The Hachette Speakers Bureau provides a wide range of authors for speaking events. To find out more, go to www.hachettespeakersbureau.com or call (866) 376-6591.

Library of Congress Cataloging-in-Publication Data

Names: Sadeghi, Habib, author.
Title: The clarity cleanse : 12 Steps to finding renewed energy, spiritual fulfillment, and emotional healing / Habib Sadeghi, DO, FACEMIP ; foreword by Gwyneth Paltrow.
Description: New York : Grand Central Life & Style, [2017]
Identifiers: LCCN 2017031272| ISBN 9781455542246 (hardcover) | ISBN 9781478923701 (audio download) | ISBN 9781455542239 (ebook)
Subjects: LCSH: Mental healing. | Emotions. | Spiritual life. | Well-being.
Classification: LCC RZ400 .S195 2017 | DDC 615.8/528—dc23
LC record available at https://lccn.loc.gov/2017031272

ISBNs: 978-1-4555-4222-2 (trade paperback), 978-1-4555-4223-9 (ebook)

Printed in the United States of America

LSC-C

10 9 8 7 6 5 4 3 2 1

To the memory of my brother, H. Mehrdad Sadeghi, MD, and innumerable other trailblazers in the field of free thinking

"Every smallest step in the field of free thinking, and of the personally formed life, has ever been fought for at the cost of spiritual and physical tortures...change has required its innumerable martyrs...nothing has been bought more dearly than that little bit of human reason & sense of freedom that is now the basis of our pride."

—*Friedrich Nietzsche,*
The Day of Dawn *(1881)*

Contents

Foreword

by Gwyneth Paltrow

In his very first piece for goop, Dr. Habib Sadeghi wrote about the truth—and why it's so difficult to tell it. His wasn't the standard definition of lying; he was talking about how we have collectively been raised to prioritize politeness over personal integrity, that we have been raised to believe that skirting the truth and covering it up with white lies is a better path forward than speaking straight. He clarifies that ignoring our feelings is not only dishonest, but that refusing to honor and give voice to them is the most harmful kind of dishonesty there is.

When I first started seeing Dr. Sadeghi many years ago, it was for some seemingly unrelated medical issues—but before he got to the medicine, he made me address the idea of living honestly. He believes that disease takes root when we are not living authentically, and not taking care of our emotional waste. He traced what was happening in my ovaries to my thyroid, otherwise known as the throat chakra—a common source of affliction for many women who do not feel empowered to speak, who stuff and stifle emotional pain rather than speaking the truth out of their mouth.

When I first met Dr. Sadeghi, I believed that honesty was a way of acting or a mindset. I now understand that it is something far deeper. It is giving yourself the space to actually feel your feelings and be true to them, at all costs. Dr. Sadeghi has become a mentor in many capacities for me, though most notably for teaching me how to live in a way that is honest. It has been one of the most beautiful, painful, and interesting lessons of my life.

As you will discover in these pages, Dr. Sadeghi brings much clarity to every aspect of living—and with clarity, comes healing.

Love,
GP

Preface

While modern medicine has many benefits, it's clear to most of us that it also has its limits. For all the advanced technology and billions of dollars poured into research each year, our approach to illness is mostly ineffective when it comes to curing chronic diseases and neurodegenerative disorders, in fact, many diseases. While diagnostics have greatly improved over the last 60 or so years, how we end up treating the diseases we diagnose has in many ways remained essentially the same.

It's clear that if healthcare is to avoid stagnation and evolve to meet the challenges of the future, in addition to the diseases we've been dealing with for more than a century, we need to think about disease differently. We must reframe our understanding of everything from what disease is and why it occurs to how we interact with it. Given our aging population and the prevalence of chronic illness, we have no choice. We simply must find a way of approaching illness that goes beyond just surgery and drugs, or our children's children will find themselves facing the same chronic killers their great-great-grandparents faced.

To think in this way requires going against many of the established, institutionalized ideas we have about biology and medicine. It means we must dare to question the unquestionable. There may even be sacred cows that, at risk of being called a nutcase or quack, should be called into question—an approach that, in countless areas of medicine, proved to be the key to major advances. If medicine is to move forward, we must become trailblazers in a profession where stepping even slightly outside the accepted lines can mean the loss of one's reputation and even one's career. Still, it's a path we must tread if humanity and medicine are to progress.

Without question, the catalyst behind every great discovery of human civilization, especially with regard to science and medicine, has proved to be intuition. It's the internal conviction, the inexplicable knowing, that possesses a researcher and convinces such an individual that the particle, process, energetic principle, or cure they are searching for actually exists, even in the face of no physical evidence or prior research. It's the ability to see the unseen before it becomes obvious to everyone else, along with resisting the urging of naysayers to be "realistic" and live within the limits of what we can experience with our senses.

Only a person with an all-consuming intuitive drive and a fearless spirit can manifest the possible from the impossible and thereby change the way we experience life. Ignaz Semmelweis, a 19th-century physician, was just such a person. He firmly believed that an invisible factor, which we today commonly refer to as bacteria, was behind the deaths of thousands of expectant mothers. He insisted that the simple act of washing hands before either performing surgery or delivering babies could greatly reduce patient deaths from infection and puerperal fever. Initially he was mercilessly humiliated by the medical establishment, even losing his job for suggesting something that's now common practice. Today the largest university in Hungary is named after him.

In the 1860s, Russian chemist Dimitri Mendeleev created the Periodic Table of Elements, which organized all the physical building blocks of the universe into a cohesive logical order. The table included the elements gold, silver, lead, argon, neon, helium, and every other known mineral, metal, and gas at the time. While the table was incredibly helpful to science, it had a problem. Wherever Mendeleev couldn't find a transitional substance that connected two elements already on the table, he left the space between them blank. While his table worked well for certain kinds of research, his detractors were quick to point out the gaps in the chart. At that time, there were no known elements with the right atomic weights to fill those spaces and complete the chart so that it made sense. When questioned about these gaps, Mendeleev stated that while the holes in the chart did exist, it wasn't proof the corresponding elements didn't. He simply said we had to continue searching.

Down to the minutest detail, Mendeleev intuited the presence of elements for which there was no tangible evidence of their existence. Today every one of those elements has indeed been discovered and Mendeleev's table is complete. He bequeathed to us a perfect example of how staying focused on the bigger picture and not getting hung up on the finer details is what brings a vision into being. Just because we don't have proof that something exists doesn't mean it isn't there.

In 1865, German chemist Friedrich August Kekulé had a dream in which he saw atoms dancing around and linking to each other. Upon awakening, he followed his intuition and immediately sketched the image he had seen in his dream. In a further dream, he saw the atoms dance around, then form circular strings that appeared to simulate a snake eating its own tail. Instead of doubting the dream, he went with his gut instinct. Kekulé was to discover that his nighttime images were a near-perfect match for the chemical composition and cyclic nature of benzene.

Semmelweis, Mendeleev, and Kekulé trusted their intuition, believed in the unseen, and were proven right. Today there's an equally powerful and invisible force at play in chronic illness that has yet to be recognized and incorporated into treatment. That force is consciousness.

Human consciousness varies from person to person but is made up of the thoughts and feelings, both conscious and unconscious, we experience regarding everything from our job to our relationships and the world around us with respect to how we feel about ourselves. Each one of us lives within our own energetic frequency, which is self-generated by individual thoughts and feelings. It's this frequency that permeates every cell of the body and plays a major role in its physical expression, whether that be health, disease, or something in between.

At the same time, our personal frequencies are interacting with the energetic frequencies of other people and even the earth itself to create the collective energetic frequency of the planet on which all living things exist. It's this collective energy, which we all draw from and interact with, that I call the "field." Like fish in the sea, consciousness moves in, around, and through us, impacting our lives every day. Not only do we interact with it, we simultaneously create it individually and collectively.

It's by accessing this unseen energy through our thoughts, then charging it in either a positive or negative way based on our feelings, that we influence our cells to develop in either healthy or diseased ways.

The idea that we develop our body and create our state of health or illness from unseen energy might seem strange at first glance—until we realize that creating physical matter from unseen energy happens all around us every day. A seed placed in the earth absorbs water, germinates, and sprouts. The sprout needs nothing but invisible energy from the sun to engage in photosynthesis and the production of carbon dioxide, a gas that's also invisible, for it to grow its thin and fragile body into a massive tree. In fact the trunk and leaves of a tree contain little of the trace minerals from the soil in which it's rooted. A tree literally creates its physical body out of thin air, utilizing the unseen energetic forces we know exist and yet cannot experience with our senses. In much the same way, we also create our physical bodies from the invisible energy of the field.

So when someone receives a medical diagnosis that informs them they have disease X, that the survival statistics are Y, and that the best treatment is Z, we're dealing only in the concrete world of physical matter—the world of effects that arise from the elements of the unseen world, which in the final analysis is the energy of the field. It stands to reason then that if we are to truly heal disease, we must look beyond matter and beyond individual parts to the world of energy where thoughts and emotions created a negative frequency that eventually manifested as a diseased body.

Much of the current medical model is trapped in the concrete world, the world of effects, unaware there's an entire unseen world of energy from which everything we observe is created. This leaves even the world's most brilliant researchers sometimes chasing red herrings, while all the while imagining they are going to find the cause of physical diseases in the physical world, when the reality is that the opposite is often the case.

The approach is so reductionist that it continues to break the human body down into its thousands of separate parts, right down to the tiniest physical components such as molecules and atoms. And still we fail to find either the cause of or cure for chronic disease, which of course we never will because it doesn't lie in our physicality.

With the understanding we have today, we can dissect a bird down to its smallest components, yet we'll never be able to observe the forces that enable it to fly. The miracle of flight only happens through the synergy of a bird's parts. Similarly, we can't discover what makes water wet by tearing the molecules apart. Hydrogen and oxygen are gasses that have entirely different properties from water.

It's only when we examine and experience them together that moisture enters the picture.

Rationalists have a problem with the intuitive aspect of healing and insist on tearing the bird or the human body into ever-smaller parts, while in the process destroying that which they are attempting to heal. In the case of some diseases, it's understood but unspoken in the medical community that it's often the "cure" that kills the patient long before the disease. There are many examples where the reductionist approach of treating separate body parts through surgery or medication, instead of regarding the whole patient as a mind-body system, only makes things worse.

It's been said that if you do what you've always done, you'll get the same outcome you've always gotten. After more than 100 years of treating chronic illnesses with drugs and surgery with no cure in sight, is it time to consider whether the traditional approach needs to change? Surely it's incumbent upon every physician who takes healing seriously to consider whether a more integrative understanding of healing that incorporates the patient's state of consciousness into the process is needed at this time.

Of course, this would mean taking a more intuitive approach to healthcare, which would result in a broader understanding of how the healing process works. It would mean being aware of what we don't know and being okay with this. Needless to say, admitting we don't have answers can be difficult for physicians, given our deep commitment to helping patients who are suffering.

While certain physical symptoms and issues must be addressed with physical treatment, lasting healing, not mere symptom management, requires a shift in perspective from being preoccupied with the concrete aspects of disease to recognizing the larger and often abstract forces underlying the whole process.

Instead of only looking for which prescription or procedure can address a physical problem, as a patient you might ask yourself,

"What is my body trying to say to me through this experience? What is it in my emotional world that might be contributing to this disease in my physical world? What is there that I can address in my energetic or emotional body to support the intervention my doctor is implementing in my physical body?"

This is what it means to achieve clarity. It requires an understanding of the deeper, unseen, and energetic psycho-spiritual aspects of the disease process as they pertain to your life, then consciously interacting with the energetic field both in and around the body to change the way it manifests physically in terms of your health. Because clarity works at the emotional and spiritual level, more than anything else it's a mindset, the effects of which eventually appear in the body.

When it comes to healing, the individual who has the disease is far more important than the disease itself, since every person's energetic frequency is unique and manifests in their body in its own way based on their history, relationships, and emotional state. Eventually everyone's biography becomes their biology. So it's not about being diagnosed, getting the same treatment everyone else gets, and expecting it to work differently for you. It's about discovering why the illness manifested in you, in which particular part of the body it appeared, how your state of consciousness or personal energetic frequency played a role in it, and how doing the work to assist your body in healing by addressing your unresolved and often unconscious emotional issues helps create your personal cure.

This is why intuition is just as important, if not more so, than any procedure you have or medication you may take. It's the unseen world of energy and emotion that creates the physical, and never the other way around. Because of this we can rebuild our own bodies with the energy of thoughts and emotions by interacting with the larger energy field around us, just as a sprout transforms its body into a tree from nothing more than the unseen energies around it.

Paracelsus, who is revered in modern medicine and considered the Father of Toxicology, himself said, "The spirit is the master, imagination the tool, and the body the plastic material. The power of the imagination is a great factor in medicine. It may produce diseases in man and in animal, and it may cure them…ills of the body may be cured by physical remedies or by the power of the spirit acting through the soul."

Can you imagine a doctor saying this to a patient in their examining room? And yet much of modern medical theory is based on the ideas of Paracelsus. Perhaps following our intuition and using imagination, emotion, and energy to facilitate healing, in addition to treating the body, isn't so crazy after all. In fact, no drug exists that can compete with the healing power of imagination and the energy it produces.

The way I have chosen to simultaneously treat a patient's mind and body is through a process I created called Integrative Psycho-Synthesis (iPs). Through one-on-one exploration and prescribed exercises, I assist patients in recognizing and resolving emotional issues, many decades old or even long forgotten, that contribute significantly to their dis-*ease* process. The patient works with the energy within him- or herself, as well as with the larger field, to alter patterns of thought and emotion, thereby generating a new frequency that's supportive of healing and initiates the anabolic process of rejuvenation.

In a very real sense, iPs is the photosynthesis of human consciousness, where we draw what we need to renew ourselves from the invisible energy within and around us. This involves much more than merely visualizing a healthy body. It's about recognizing and releasing a way of thinking and being that hasn't only become detrimental but unconsciously addictive.

Because each person's circumstances are different, what's more important than the fact that they became sick is *why* they became sick. In the future of medicine, the personal life context that precedes a patient's illness will be just as important, if not more so, in the healing process as treating the physical aspects of the disease. Context is far more important than content when it comes to health.

So while it can be scary to get a serious diagnosis, I do my best to focus my patients on doing the deeper work rather than being preoccupied with the physical details of their illness. How we choose to relate to the issue of disease is the real issue for both doctor and patient, and it's only by working together in this way that we'll finally defeat the most serious diseases of our time.

I've seen hundreds of patients make miraculous recoveries from illnesses that were considered incurable by doing this kind of work. Some of their stories you'll read in this book. I owe my own recovery from cancer over 20 years ago to techniques I discovered through following my intuition. These techniques, together with additional interventions I developed while earning my master's degree in spiritual psychology with an emphasis in consciousness, health and healing at the University of Santa Monica is the program offered here.

There have been times when an incredulous patient has asked me, "How do you know this works? Why should I bother? Where's the research?"

I know this works because I'm alive more than 20 years later, with no chemotherapy or radiation. I know this works because of the patients I've seen transformed before my very eyes over a few short years, and sometimes even months. No evidence can be more convincing than when dramatic healing power touches your life in a personal way.

You may be tempted to dismiss such cases as anecdotal, a fluke, as if to imply that one person is somehow more special than another and has some secret power that everyone else doesn't possess. This is simply a fear-based reaction that seeks to dismiss anything we can't fully explain or understand. But as great men and women of science have demonstrated again and again, just because we can't explain or even see something doesn't mean it isn't real.

If you're looking for volumes of research confirming the healing connection between the mind and body, you won't find it here or likely anywhere, given that nearly all research is funded by pharmaceutical corporations for which, if there's no financial incentive to develop a treatment for a particular illness and thus make a profit from it, it's largely ignored. Why focus on a more holistic way of healing when there are billions in profit to be made from managing the symptoms of diseases with lifelong medication, rather than curing those diseases outright?

If you're the kind of person who needs proof that this or that will work, with a guarantee of a specific outcome, you might consider the fact that even traditional allopathic medicine can't provide that kind of promise. If, however, you're the kind of patient who intuitively feels you might possess more healing power than you thought, even though you don't know how to access it, and are the kind of person who takes a proactive approach to your health instead of expecting the doctor to simply fix what's wrong the same way a mechanic fixes your car, there is much here that may well change your life.

What's required at the outset is the suspension of disbelief and being open to the possibilities. When we attend the theater, in order to have an immersive experience we don't have to understand, and may not care to understand lest they lose their magic, how all the special effects are achieved behind the scenes. In fact, the less we fixate on the finer details and instead focus our attention on the bigger picture and larger action that's unfolding on the stage in front of us, the richer and more real the experience will be.

I encourage you to follow your intuition and step into the unknown, understanding that you don't need all the answers. You just need to do your part. You are not alone on this journey, as many have come before you and achieved great success because, like you, they intuitively understood that healing isn't simply a matter of a prescription or surgical procedure. It involves a way of perceiving yourself through trust, possibility, and most of all clarity.

Upon this age, that never speaks its mind,
This furtive age, this age endowed with power
To wake the moon with footsteps, fit an oar
Into the rowlocks of the wind, and find
What swims before his prow, what swirls behind—
Upon this gifted age, in its dark hour,
Falls from the sky a meteoric shower
Of facts . . . they lie unquestioned, uncombined.

Wisdom enough to leech us of our ill
Is daily spun; but there exists no loom
To weave it into fabric; undefiled
Proceeds pure Science, and has her say; but still
Upon this world from the collective womb
Is spewed all day the red triumphant child.
　　　　　—Edna St. Vincent Millay, "Huntsman, What Quarry?"

Awakening to Clarity

In 1955 a massive Buddha encrusted with thousands of bits of colored glass was in the process of being relocated to a new pagoda at the temple of Wat Traimit in Bangkok, Thailand. This was no easy task, considering the 200-year-old statue stood nearly ten feet tall and weighed more than five tons. After several failed attempts to lift the mass from its pedestal, workers tried again, only to watch helplessly as support ropes broke and the statue came crashing to the ground. Rushing to survey the damage, workers and monks were astonished at what they found. The statue was badly damaged, but only on its surface. As they peered through the cracks, they saw gold gleaming beneath.

Further investigation would show that the entire statue was originally made of gold. Its covering of plaster and glass had been added in the 18th century to hide its value and prevent it from being stolen by the invading Burmese. The secret of what lay beneath the Buddha's surface was so well kept that it had eventually been lost to history. At the time the statue was being moved, no one at the temple knew its true nature until the accident happened to reveal it.

That, in essence, is what this book is about. We all know what it's like to be lifted up, only to be dropped back down again unexpectedly, leaving us feeling cracked and damaged, possibly beyond repair.

When we're in pain, we tend to focus on the cause of that pain, which can be any number of things—illness, divorce, loss of a loved one, a difficult relationship, feeling trapped in a dead-end job, feeling depressed, finding ourselves all alone, and so many other challenges. What we often overlook is that the issue itself is never as important as how we *relate* to it. You see, any ailment, any problem, any negative experience presents us with a choice. We can choose to see our circumstances as unfortunate, ourselves as broken. Or we can choose to look past the surface damage to the gold beneath—gold we previously didn't know was there.

This life-changing shift in consciousness requires what I call *clarity*. My path to clarity came in the form of cancer.

My Wake-Up Call

I was in my second year of medical school and had just finished yet another long day of coursework. No sooner had I returned to my room than I felt the strong pull of my bed. All I wanted to do was sleep. Instead of reviewing my notes from the lecture I'd just attended, I tossed my books on the floor and my head hit my pillow. I was out cold in a matter of moments.

At 2:00 a.m., I sat straight up in bed completely awake and aware. I'd heard a voice in my head as clearly as if someone had spoken to me from across the room. It said, "Check yourself." I can't explain why, but I immediately went to the bathroom to examine my groin. There it was, on my left testicle, a lump.

For the next four hours I scoured the internet looking for every conceivable explanation for my condition. After scaring myself to death with too much information, I called my brother Mehrdad, a physician in San Diego, who tried to calm me by reminding me that medical students are notorious hypochondriacs. But I knew what was happening to me wasn't "all in my head." This was something serious—I was sure of it.

The first thing I did was seek medical insurance, which I didn't have because as a student I couldn't afford it. With the help of my brother I obtained coverage and went straight to the doctor. The diagnosis came soon after, stage-three testicular cancer with a 70 percent chance of metastasis (meaning that it would spread throughout my body).

When I heard the news and saw the doctor's report detailing how bad things already were, and how much worse they could become following treatment, especially if there were complications, my mind latched on to the information like it was the only thing in the world. This was 1997, when Olympic figure skating champion Scott Hamilton and cyclist Lance Armstrong were making headlines because of their battle with the same type of cancer. I remember being panic-stricken as I read an interview with Armstrong in which he detailed how his cancer had spread from his testicles to his lymph nodes, lungs, and brain.

My oncologists gave me only one treatment option—have my testicle removed, along with all the lymph nodes in my gut (a 16-hour procedure), followed by extensive rounds of radiation and chemotherapy, accompanied by prescriptions for anxiety and depression. The plan was so invasive that I couldn't help but wonder whether it was the best one for me. I knew it didn't feel right, but I also had no idea what "right" really meant in this extreme situation.

· ·

EXCERPTS FROM CITY OF HOPE NATIONAL MEDICAL
CENTER AND BECKMAN RESEARCH INSTITUTE, REPORT
OF SADEGHI, HABIB, MARCH 1997

· ·

This gentleman with embryonal carcinoma and vascular invasion has roughly a 70% chance of having micrometastases to the retroperitoneal lymph nodes...

Risk of infertility…

High chance of recurrence within the next year…

Would necessitate approximately four cycles of platinum-based chemotherapy…

FINAL RECOMMENDATIONS

I recommended to this patient that he undergo a left template nerve sparing retroperitoneal lymph node dissection within the next month.

We went on to talk about potential risks and complications of surgery, including but not limited to blood loss, risk of a reaction to anesthesia, abscess formation, wound infection, deep venous thrombosis, and pulmonary embolism and death.

Taking a Step Back

After the doctor handed me my diagnosis, I didn't know where to go or what to do. I felt aimless, helpless, and hopeless. Somehow I found my way to the anatomy lab at school. I don't know whether it was the overwhelming emotions or the stench of the formaldehyde that did it, but as soon as I walked in the door my eyes welled up. That was when an angel appeared to me in the form of my anatomy partner, Gary.

Gary took one look at me and said, "You're not doing well."

"I was just diagnosed with cancer," I told him.

He paused for a moment to take in this information. Then without missing a beat he suggested, "Let's go get lunch."

Gary is older than I am. At the time he was already married with a son and had a PhD in psychology. Since I looked up to and trusted him, when he proposed we eat lunch I agreed even though food was the last thing on my mind. We crossed the street to a Mexican restaurant.

As we sat across the table from each other, Gary asked me, *How are you holding up? What are you feeling? What's going on in your head?*

I was numb. It felt like an elephant-sized weight was crushing my chest and it was hard to breathe. Everything just felt wrong. Since I was so tired I could barely think, I had no idea how to figure out what I should do. Yet although I found it difficult to form the first words, as soon as I started speaking the answers poured out of me.

Gary listened as I unloaded, watching me intently with his warm hazel eyes. When I was finished, he assured me he understood. Then he said something that changed everything for me. "I don't know what God you believe in, but the God I believe in is a loving God." Pausing for a moment as he leaned in closer and looked me straight in the eye, he continued, "You're going to be okay. I don't know what that means exactly, but you're going to be okay."

Something about the way he spoke those words made me instantly believe him. It was almost like magic. The weight lifted from my chest. I felt a surge of energy. Almost without realizing it, I raised my hand to signal the waiter. Gary and I sat together in near silence as I inhaled not one, not two, but three fish tacos.

That conversation was a turning point for me. Soon after, I realized I had options when it came to treating my cancer. I realized I could say no to my doctors' plan, or at least no to most of it. I realized I could choose to keep searching for an answer that felt right for me.

That was what I did. I chose to have the testicle where I'd found the lump removed but forgo the rest of the recommended treatment. I didn't make the decision lightly and it's not one I would advocate for everyone. But after thorough research and consultation with other professionals, I knew as a medical student it was the right choice for me. Even so, my family didn't understand. My doctors thought I was insane, but I'd made up my mind. I decided to surrender to the power that seemed to know more about this situation than I did, to the voice that had told me to check myself in the first place, to the loving God Gary had reminded me of. I sensed that to surrender was to make room in my life for the answer to show up.

I knew I still needed to heal, so following the procedure to remove my testicle I took a year off medical school and went on a journey of discovery. I began in Mexico, where I studied with *curanderos*, or native healers. I backpacked my way to Guadalajara and Córdoba, Veracruz, to learn more ancient healing techniques. I went on to Germany, where I discovered German New Medicine, which holds that cells have the capacity to retain memories just like the brain and that negative energy from unresolved emotional issues plays a significant role in creating disease. I traveled to Himachal Pradesh in Northern India, where I explored meditation, yoga, and massage, and deepened my knowledge of osteopathic medicine. I didn't receive any traditional medical treatment during this time, although I did work with various teachers to better understand myself and some of the negative feelings and misperceptions that I held.

All the while, I kept thinking about my lunch with Gary. Every morning when I awakened, I wrote the word *love* on the inside length of my thumb to remind me of the conversation we had and to give comfort whenever I grew nervous about the path I had chosen. I knew what Gary had done for me was important, but I still had questions. I especially wanted to understand how, during the course of one short conversation, I had gone from feeling exhausted, overwhelmed, helpless, and hopeless, to feeling energized, assured...and hungry. How had that been possible?

Over time I came to understand that what Gary had done for me was to shine a light of clarity on my darkest moment. He provided me with a way to contain my emotions. He gave credence and context to the thoughts and feelings that were clogging my being—the fear that was sapping my energy, the overwhelming emotions that were manifesting as a weight on my chest, the powerlessness that was killing my appetite. This allowed me to look past these things to the bigger picture—the sense that a loving God was looking out for me, and so in one way or another I was going to be okay.

Being able to move past my negative feelings to focus on that one comforting thought resulted in a tremendous energy shift that profoundly affected my mental and physical wellbeing. The more I learned from the teachers I met on my journey, the more I understood about the mind-body connection, which turned out to be the explanation for how, in just a few short moments, I had gone from being unable to stomach the idea of food to feeling ravenous.

I wondered whether the cancer might be a signpost pointing to something deeper within me that needed healing before my physical world could respond in kind. If so, I would never completely heal from my illness unless I first discovered how my mind and spirit were fueling it.

As I sought to understand where this signpost was pointing, I began recalling the various traumas of my childhood.

Following the Signs

Growing up in Iran can be difficult in the best of circumstances. Mine were far from perfect. Some of my earliest memories include recurring household violence and sexual abuse by a family member I loved and trusted. The guilt and shame were overwhelming, and my religious upbringing led me to believe that God was punishing me. Surely I'd done something to deserve this or it wouldn't be happening to me.

When I was twelve years old my family moved to the United States, where I was immediately placed in public school. Since I didn't speak a word of English, I had no way to express my needs at school. Neither was I encouraged to speak up and express myself at home. Coupled with the abuse I had suffered, this left me feeling disempowered. Although the abuse stopped when we moved away from my abuser, I found I still couldn't assert myself in any area of my life. It was nearly impossible for me to be direct, confident, or powerful.

This was especially the case when it came to females. Although I knew my natural orientation was heterosexual, I was practically incapable of interacting with any member of the opposite sex who wasn't either one of my teachers or a family member.

Several years after arriving in the US, even though I still didn't have any friends and I continued to struggle with English, I became determined to make a real connection with someone. My chance came one day in the high school gym during one of my regular work-outs. My lifting gloves had worn out, so Mr. Kaiser, the football coach, directed me to speak with Robbie, captain of the football team, who sold extra pairs from his locker. This was just the opportunity I'd been waiting for. Prior to that day, I got an old yearbook and cut out pictures of all the football players, including Robbie, so I could practice pronouncing their names and starting up a conversation. I kept the cutouts in my wallet so I could work on my communication skills at every opportunity. Now I was finally getting a chance to make a real human connection with the most popular guy in school.

When I approached Robbie, he understood what I was asking for and told me to follow him to his locker. I couldn't believe how nice he was being and how well everything was going. As he handed me the gloves, saying they'd be $10, I opened my wallet...whereupon all the players' photos fell out.

As Robbie looked down at the images scattered across the locker-room floor, he took a step back from me. I realized instantly that he had jumped to the wrong conclusion.

After a long pause he looked up at me and said, "Oh my God, you're a faggot." I had never heard the word before, so I didn't fully understand what he was saying, although his rejection came through in the way he said it. But with my limited English, how was I to explain the truth to him? I was in no position to counter the prejudice he displayed.

Following this incident I would have given anything to go back to being isolated and invisible. Instead I became a target. Girls would suggestively present themselves to me. When I didn't react because I believed in respecting women, they'd mockingly say to each other, "See, I told you he was queer." Boys too would say all sorts of things I didn't understand until I repeated them to Coach Kaiser. This was when I learned many of the epithets people use to shame or ridicule someone who's gay.

This was the 1980s, in the midst of the AIDS crisis and at a time when homosexuality was viewed with widespread suspicion and greater condemnation than it is today. These experiences only compounded my struggle to access my masculinity and personal power. As far as I was concerned, I was weak and ineffectual. People had abused me my entire life and it seemed like this was the way it would always be.

Breaking Through

The insight I've shared concerning my earlier life came to the surface during my travels and studies of alternative forms of healing. All of this provided me with a new perspective on my illness. I understood that although *I* couldn't lead the charge to fight the cancer within me, *it* could lead *me*. For this to happen, I needed to go within myself and see what my cancer was trying to tell me.

Based on everything I'd learned, it struck me as no coincidence that years of sexual abuse, repressed emotions, sexual humiliation in high school, and struggles with assertiveness and masculinity had created negative energy that manifested as cancer in my sexual organs.

A stunning realization now came to me. The cancer wasn't trying to kill me—it was trying to bring attention to the fact that I had adopted some serious misperceptions about myself and my world. I had accepted a negative view of myself and was living as if it were the truth, not a faulty belief that could be altered. What's more, I'd been doing this for so long that it had made me sick.

I finally heard the message my cancer had been trying to tell me. I had to start seeing myself for who I really was, seeing the world for what it really was—and I had to do these things without blame or judgment, which would only serve as a distraction.

I also saw that I had to bring this kind of clarity to both my past experiences and my present ones. After all, it wasn't just the childhood traumas that I was struggling with. My choice to remove the testicle where a cancerous tumor had been found brought back those old insecurities about my masculinity. Worse yet, I was told it would make it nearly impossible for me to father children, a verdict that I found profoundly difficult to accept, worrying that it made me less of a man and meant no woman would want to settle down with me.

After my travels I continued to go for regular checkups with my doctors at City of Hope, the renowned cancer hospital and research center near Los Angeles. Although the malignancy had been removed, my blood panels still showed markers for cancer. Would the disease return, possibly in a different area of my body? If so, when?

Despite the unknowns, I continued to reject any further medical intervention, focusing instead on increasing my clarity and inhabiting more of my authentic self. As I pursued this course, I knew something was changing. I couldn't explain it, but I could feel it.

Eighteen months after first finding the lump, I got a call from a friend who ran a lab where I'd sent a sample of my blood. He knew my story, which was why he called me personally. He could hardly contain his excitement as he said, "Habib, there are no biomarkers for cancer here. You really are cancer-free!" This was it—proof of the energetic shift I had been experiencing.

Soon after this call I saw my oncologist for a follow-up test and examination. It was true. I was cancer-free and remain so to this day.

I even have the City of Hope paperwork to prove it. I'm also happy to say that, despite what I had been told about the unlikelihood of fathering children, I went on to marry a wonderful woman who accepted me in spite of those predictions, and together we have two wonderful children conceived the old-fashioned way.

And that's not all. In the years since becoming cancer-free, I finished my medical degree and, together with my wife, Dr. Sherry Sami, started a thriving medical practice in Los Angeles, where I have helped thousands of patients not only heal physically but also emotionally, mentally, and spiritually by showing them how to find clarity.

In 1997, when I had that life-changing conversation with Gary on the day of my diagnosis, he had planted a seed that directed my focus to the word *love*. It became like a mantra to me, an idea that I would contemplate each day until years later my wife and I started the Love Button Global Movement with the mission to educate and empower people to transform their communities through loving acts of kindness (LoveButton.org). It was even highlighted in Super Bowl 50 when the band Coldplay, led by singer Chris Martin, supplied all 75,000 attendees with their own Love Buttons to wear. During their halftime show, they also had the entire stadium hold up colored placards for all the world to see—an estimated 111 million television viewers. The placards bore the message Believe in Love. It was an inspiring tribute to what clarity can do because, as you'll soon learn, having more clarity leads to having more love in your life.

What Clarity Can Do for You

By learning how to create clarity for myself, I was finally able to consciously create *a life that was worthy of me.*

Most importantly, I discovered that living with clarity didn't require finding something or adding something to myself that I didn't already possess. I had everything I needed, we all do. I just didn't know this until I learned to see who I was and what was happening to me from a new perspective. Because my illness is what led me to this shift in consciousness, I never say I had cancer. I say I had *canswer*.

My parents weren't literate. My dad worked in a service station and my mom babysat to earn enough to care for my two brothers and me. Clearly it wasn't my background that enabled me to achieve my dreams. On the contrary, I owe everything to clarity. The fact I've been able to transcend the cultural, economic, and language barriers of my upbringing, as well as move beyond my emotional traumas and a serious illness in order to finish my medical degree, become a doctor, and start my own practice, is in my mind a testament to the power of clarity.

Of course, I didn't get here all at once. A decade after all I had learned following my diagnosis, I found myself working as the assistant medical director of the largest occupational medicine clinic in California. Every day I saw people who had been injured at work, with conditions as common as lower back pain or as uncommon as having a finger cut off by machinery. It was important work, but the environment I was in wasn't one that truly fostered healing. I saw upward of 60 patients a day, spending no more than twelve minutes per person, rushing patients through as if I were working on an assembly line.

Speed was the priority, and this orientation spilled over into my personal life. When my wife spoke to me I hurried her along, prompting her to get to the point. Then, one day while driving too fast on the freeway, I was in a car accident. This was the crisis that brought me back to clarity. To help myself heal from the accident, I went on a ten-day meditation retreat where I had an epiphany that I needed to change the way I was living my life, including the way I worked. I rented a 350-square-foot office and hung out my shingle. My medical practice was born and in six months I was booked solid.

That has been my journey so far. The rest of this book will be about yours. As it was for me, growth and progress may not have followed a straight line in your life, and you may currently be feeling stuck, unfulfilled, or even as if you're moving backward. Clarity can make all the difference, as it has for the thousands of patients I have helped heal not only physically but also emotionally, mentally, and spiritually.

People typically first come to me because of some physical ailment, with complaints ranging from hair loss and weight management problems to autoimmune disease and advanced-stage cancer. While I use traditional treatment options to help my patients, I also go well beyond this to alleviate their suffering. No matter the physical ailment, it can always be traced back to something deeper.

Because illness is an expression, a symptom, of a deeper wound, I spend considerable time familiarizing myself with all the different aspects of my patients' lives. Without exception, I have been able to trace the cause of their condition back to a lack of clarity. The circumstances that caused this lack are different for each person, but it's through finding their way back to clarity that they heal. Consequently my practice involves teaching people the path to clarity. It's how I not only help my patients get better but empower them to go on to live healthier, happier, more fulfilling lives.

The knowledge I've gained and the methods I've adopted since the onset of my illness can help anyone who's living an unfulfilled life. This lack of fulfillment may manifest itself in the form of illness, but it might just as easily be expressed as feeling stuck, blocked, uninspired, anxious, disconnected, disempowered, depressed, or more often than not a combination of several of these all at once. Regardless of the symptoms or condition, clarity is the key to addressing *any* problem. Clarity is what provides the framework for healing emotionally, healing physically, becoming empowered, letting go of stress and negative energy, and ultimately leading the life we were always meant to lead.

To do this, you don't need to learn to love yourself, think posi-tively, or accomplish any of the other goals espoused by the New Age movement. Quite the opposite, achieving clarity requires honoring all your emotions—the positive, the negative, and the in-between. By honoring them, you integrate them into the clear space inside you that's your true being. Once integrated, they empower you to both discover and express the power, perfection, and love you already are.

Clarity is what allows all of us to recognize the painful events of our lives as golden opportunities to throw off limitations, inhabit our authentic selves, and expand our lives in ways that wouldn't have been possible without the experiences we go through. Then, like the golden Buddha, we can shed our dull, limiting disguise and open ourselves up to a better, brighter, more powerful experience of the world.

I invite you to start doing that with me right now.

THE LAW OF LIFE

Love Begets Love,
Love Creates Life,
Life cultivates suffering,
Suffering whispers fear,
Fear accompanies Courage,
Courage Carries Confidence,
Confidence whispers Hope,
Hope Gives Life,
Life invites Love,
Love Begets Love.
    —Dr. Habib Sadeghi (with help from Margot Bickel)

PART I

GETTING CLEAR ON CLARITY

CHAPTER ONE

What Is Clarity?

When people ask me what it means to have clarity, I ask them to imagine themselves making a cup of tea. What do you need to make tea? The answers I usually get are hot water and, of course, tea leaves.

These two things are certainly necessary for making tea, but they aren't the only requirements. They aren't even the most important. When making tea, the first thing you need, before anything else, is a cup. You need a container in which to place the tea leaves and pour the water.

Clarity is that cup. The experiences we have and the things we do are the tea leaves and water that go into the cup. Together they can make a wonderfully tasty and nourishing tea, but it doesn't work unless you have a cup. Imagine what would happen if you tried to make tea without a cup. When you poured water over your tea leaves, there would be nothing to contain them, so you wouldn't get a nice cup of tea at all. All you would get would be a mess.

Like lacking a cup, lacking clarity is no small matter. Without it we are unable to contain or give context to our actions and the things that happen in our lives. It's why so many of us are unsure of what

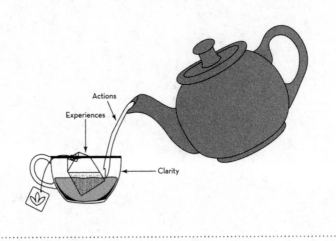

to do when we feel stuck or unhappy. It's why we feel unprepared for life's challenges and traumatic events.

When I was in medical school, I memorized a phone book's worth of information each week, but none of it taught me anything about how to live my life. That's why, when I received my cancer diagnosis, I was lost. I knew a lot about cancer and how it affected the body, but I had no idea how to handle the fact that I was now facing it myself. Like water being poured over tea leaves without a cup, my thoughts and feelings flowed all over the place. I was a mess—until, that is, my friend Gary came along and did for me what I couldn't do for myself. He contained me. In that crucial moment, he served as my cup.

Without this tremendous gift that Gary gave me, I don't believe I would have been able to heal from cancer. That lunch in the Mexican restaurant was the start of my recovery. Later on I realized I needed to be able to do for myself what Gary had done for me. Cancer was my challenge of the moment, but it wasn't going to be the only difficulty I would face. I couldn't go through life hoping Gary, or someone as generous and knowledgeable, would be around every time I needed clarity. I had to learn how to serve as my own container—how to create my own cup.

A potter creates a cup by knowing which parts of the clay to keep and which to discard as she forms her vessel. In much the same way, clarity is what allows us to take from any experience the lessons we can use—those elements that help us learn, grow, and expand our consciousness. Then we discard the rest, continually clearing our cup of all the fear, resentment, judgment, sadness, and other bits and pieces that won't serve us moving forward. Such things only get in our way, and perhaps even harm us, when we allow them to stick around.

The Theory of Containment

Clarity has its roots in a theory developed in the 1960s by British psychoanalyst Wilfred Bion. The basic idea behind Bion's theory is that, in order for us to process our thoughts and feelings fully and effectively, we must first be able to *contain* them. This is the opposite of what most of us instinctively do with uncomfortable or unhappy feelings, which is to ignore, dismiss, or try to change or control them.

Containing means being able to gather and hold what we're feeling, being present with it so that we consciously experience it in a nonjudgmental and empathic way. As we process it in this way, we enable it to pass through us.

Ironically it's this containment, this act of holding, that allows us to *move through* our thoughts and emotions. It's a process that both requires space and creates space.

To understand what I mean, think about cleaning house. A few years ago hoarding became a popular subject for the cable networks. A&E had a show called *Hoarders*, TLC had *Hoarding: Buried Alive*, and the Style Network featured ten seasons of *Clean House*. If you've seen any of these shows, or know someone who hoards, you know the mess hoarders live in is something that builds up over time. It might start with a few piles of newspapers on the floor, stacks of clothes that never get put away, or dishes piling up in the sink. As hoarding habits continue, a little clutter turns into crowdedness. Then the crowdedness spreads, first across one room, then across two. If a person continues on this trajectory, pretty soon their house is overrun. In an extreme hoarder's home stacks of stuff lie everywhere, the floor is barely visible, and the hoarder has hardly any room to move. Because they haven't cleaned things up, they can't move around, which makes it hard to clean since there's no room to maneuver.

We get stuck in much the same way psychologically and spiritually, or psycho-spiritually, as I call it, when we suppress or internalize our thoughts and feelings. As the saying goes, "Feelings buried alive never die." In other words, if we don't make a habit of containing and processing our feelings and thoughts, our internal landscape goes through the same kind of devolution as that of a hoarder's house. Such feelings and thoughts hang around, cluttering up our consciousness. Over time, unaddressed clutter will continue to build, not only crowding out our authentic being but festering and becoming unsanitary, even downright dangerous. When the buildup reaches this level in our internal landscape, that's when disease erupts in our bodies or our life circumstances.

Clarity, therefore, isn't just a cup. Clarity is a clean cup. In order for our tea to be tasty, healthy, and restorative, we not only need a cup to drink from, we need that cup to be clean. Achieving clarity isn't only about creating a container but about keeping the container decongested and free from contaminants.

The muck stuck in the bottom of our cups consists of our biases and prejudices. It's our limiting beliefs and our many distractions. It's repressed emotions and unprocessed experiences (bad or good) that stick with us, drain our energy, and get in our way. We need a way to process and make sense of the things that happen in our lives—all the experiences we have, the thoughts we think, the emotions we feel—so this muck doesn't stick around and build up until it overwhelms us. Like cleaning house, this is an ongoing process. The longer we go without taking action, the more work there's going to be when we finally start, and the more likely it is we'll unearth something truly nasty that's been growing unseen in the darkness.

Thirty spokes share the wheel's hub;
It is the center hole that makes it useful.
Shape clay into a vessel;
It is the space within that makes it useful.
Cut doors and windows for a room;
It is the holes which make it useful.
Therefore benefit comes from what is there;
Usefulness from what is not there.

—Lao Tzu, *Tao Te Ching*

What a Lack of Clarity Looks Like in Everyday Life

To envision how a lack of clarity could be showing up in your everyday life, think about a couple in the midst of an argument. For them to come to a mutual understanding and proceed in a way that's best for the relationship rather than for either individual, the conversation needs a context. There needs to be agreement that the other has a valid perspective and deserves to be heard. The couple can then usually work toward a positive resolution.

However, you've doubtless not only witnessed or even been a part of disagreements that lack context and observed how quickly they can go off the rails. Voices grow louder as the two sides struggle to make themselves heard and understood. Instead of listening closely, the parties talk over one another, interrupting to try (usually unsuccessfully) to make their points.

In such a situation, both are more interested in proving who's right than in coming to a mutual understanding. Because they can't agree on what "right" is, they get stuck on repeat instead of moving forward. The language becomes harsher, more judgmental, more emotionally charged. The conversation quickly devolves into an uncontained mess, leading to anger, frustration, and hurt feelings, with no mutually satisfactory resolution in sight.

Does any of this sound familiar?

How about this one? I once saw an acquaintance's toddler, who was learning to walk, waddle unaware straight into a glass door. The little boy fell to the floor and immediately burst into tears. He wasn't injured, but he experienced a mixture of fear, confusion, and upset that his young mind didn't yet know how to process. Alerted to the situation by her child's cries, his mother hurried over to him. But instead of reaching out to comfort him, she immediately started yelling, "Oh my God, oh my God, what's happened to you?" Glancing around the room, she spied her husband, and began chiding. "Why did you leave this door closed? Why weren't you watching him? What's wrong with you!" The husband, feeling blamed and wounded, yelled back. That poor little boy, reacting to his parents' uncontained emotions, howled even louder.

Instead of reacting from a state of distress or looking for someone to blame, the mother could have contained her feelings. She could have calmly walked over and picked up her child, hugged him, wiped away his tears, and gently assured him that everything was going to be okay. Once the child had been sufficiently soothed, so that he calmed down, she might then have tapped the glass to help her son understand what had happened to him. She could have shown him how to walk past or around the glass so he wouldn't repeat his accident. In this way she could have contained his feelings and contextualized his experience, allowing him to return to emotional equilibrium and modeling how to one day do this for himself. Our parents, and especially our mothers, are our primary teachers in the art of emotional containment, but if they haven't mastered it for themselves their children may never learn it.

A lack of clarity doesn't just show up in our lives as negative experiences and difficult relationships. It can also mean the difference between life and death, as was brought home to me not long ago when I was in my car heading home on a packed Los Angeles freeway. A motorcycle zigzagged by me, threading through the crawling traffic. "Please slow down," I said out loud as I saw him come within inches of a car's bumper. Moments later, I watched in horror as another car changed lanes just ahead of him. Because the motorcyclist was moving too fast to get out of the way, he plowed right into the car. As his motorcycle crashed to the ground, I watched his body sail through the air.

I immediately pulled over and rushed to the man's side. When I got there, a woman who had been closer to the accident was already with him. This guy couldn't even move, and yet he was asking her about his motorcycle. "If I were you, I wouldn't worry about your motorcycle right now," she told him. "You're in horrible shape."

The man's eyes widened in fear when he heard this, so I decided I had better step in. Afraid he would go into shock if someone didn't contain him, I knelt down by his side, held his hand, and looked him in the eye as I said, "I'm a doctor and you've been in an accident. An ambulance is on its way. The good news is the worst is over now and you're going to heal."

When I said this, I could see the man practically melt with relief. I had his attention. To keep him present and in a state of relative calm, I kept talking. "I want to ask you some questions. I want to call someone for you. Who can I call?"

"My sister," he answered. "Her name is..."

I wrote her name down on my hand.

"Great, you're doing great. Now, do you have any allergies?"

"No."

"Do you take any medications?"

"Yes," and he listed a few. I wrote those on my hand as well.

We continued talking until the ambulance arrived. By that time, not only did I have all the information the paramedics needed, the man was calm and contained. He was no longer breathing heavily or fixated on his motorcycle. His eyes were no longer darting all over the place. Despite his injuries, he was able to engage, answer questions, and understand what was happening, which is the best state to be in to participate in your own healing.

The situation could have played out very differently. It could have been a chaotic, confusing, and frightening experience for that motorcyclist. But it wasn't, and this can make a crucial difference. Research has shown that if you walk into a traumatic situation and do what I did, you actually increase the person's chances of surviving.

In every situation we encounter, from relationships to parenting, traumatic events and beyond, clarity is what we need in order to process the situation, give it meaning, and ultimately heal emotionally, spiritually, and physically. Without clarity, life can quickly get out of hand and stay that way.

What Clarity Looks Like in Everyday Life

Having clarity means having the psycho-spiritual space we need to process and make sense of everything that happens in our lives—all the experiences we have, all the thoughts we think, all the emotions we experience. But it is so much more.

In the beginning, creating clarity may be mostly about cleaning your internal house. You may be starting out with a lot of repressed feelings and unresolved traumas or issues you need to deal with in order to clean your cup. But once it's clean and you have a process in place to help you keep it clean, you will be able to create clarity on a regular basis, which is when things change.

With clarity on your side, you'll find yourself more prepared for whatever life may throw at you. You'll better enjoy the ups and more easily handle the downs. You'll be more resilient, and more powerful, and better able to steer your life in the direction you want it to go.

When we stop blaming and judging ourselves and others, stop internalizing negative feelings and experiences, a great burden is lifted. With clarity comes a positive shift in our self-image and self-esteem. The immediate result is an expanding sense of freedom.

In this frame of mind we naturally make choices that benefit us, so that our lives start to work again. Because we're thinking of and treating ourselves differently, other people react differently to us. New opportunities arise and troubled relationships either improve or resolve in an organic way, making room for new friends, business associates, or romantic partners.

At the same time, clarity provides a powerful confidence boost. "Not enough" and "I can't" aren't obstacles any longer, so that we begin taking risks and doing things we never thought ourselves capable of or gave ourselves permission to try. Clarity provides both the joy and the courage required to live with absolutely no regrets.

I saw this shift happen with Brian, an actor who came to me because he was losing his hair. It began with his facial hair, then his eyebrows, and finally the hair atop his head. Alopecia is a difficult experience for anyone, but it was especially troubling for someone like

Brian who made his living as an actor. It wasn't just his self-esteem on the line, it was his ability to earn a living and support his family.

Various medications can treat the symptoms Brian was experiencing, but for true healing to take place we had to look beyond the prescription pad. (For the record, I'm not against many conventional methods or medications for treating disorders and disease. I just believe they are often woefully inadequate, treating the symptoms but leaving the root cause of a condition unaddressed.)

We began Brian's treatment with a conversation. As I talked with him, I discovered the hair loss that had caused him to seek my help wasn't his only symptom. He was also suffering from severe anxiety and insomnia. This suggested to me that he felt profoundly disempowered for some reason. I knew from our discussion that his marriage was quite healthy, so I asked if there had perhaps been a time in the past when he'd felt weak or powerless. As soon as I posed the question, his eyes grew wide and filled with tears. A specific incident came immediately to mind, and he began telling me about something that had happened at work.

Brian had been cast in a film that required his character to do a shower scene. Prior to going on set, he made it clear to the director that he wouldn't be removing his towel for the scene. To his relief, the director agreed to shoot around the towel until, that is, they were on set. Just as the cameras were about to start rolling, the director pointed to the towel and said gruffly, "Lose it." When Brian reminded him of their conversation, the director ignored what the actor was saying and grew increasingly impatient. Finally he yelled in front of everyone on set, "Come on, lose the damn towel! Don't be such a prude. You're holding up the entire production!"

Since everyone was staring at him, Brian's resolve faltered. In a moment of utter frustration and humiliation, he tossed the towel aside and went ahead with the scene. As he recounted the incident, he said he could still feel the shame of that moment as acutely as if it had only just happened. Although he was angry with himself for compromising his principles and allowing this man to bully him in front of everyone, the fact was that he felt helpless. What could he have done? Walk off set, losing money and burning professional bridges in the process? He'd needed that job, which meant the director had all the power.

From this point Brian found himself having trouble asserting himself in professional situations. As this happened more and more, his symptoms grew worse and worse. He hadn't made the connection before, but once he did he could see clearly that he couldn't continue to allow these kinds of situations to happen.

Brian's treatment centered on helping him reconnect with his inner assertiveness. (You'll learn how to do this work in part II, which describes the process for creating clarity.) To assist him with this, I handed him a special gold coin that I had received from my mentor Gary when I thought I was going to die from cancer. It was a gold South African Krugerrand and giving it to me had been Gary's way of helping me remember, as he put it, that "love is that gold you keep inside you."

For me this gold coin had come to symbolize the golden decision I had made not to accept my doctor's invasive treatment plan but to trust I could find a better way to heal. After sharing its significance in my life, I asked Brian to wrap his hand around the coin and visualize the center of his soul, which housed his sacred right to self-determination. He was so moved by the experience that he asked if he could keep the coin for a while as he made some changes in his life.

One Sunday about six months later, I was at a café feeding lunch to my young daughter, HannaH, when I felt someone touch my shoulder. I turned around to see Brian beaming at me. "Dr. Sadeghi, I just did something I think will make you proud," he announced. Then he told me about the short film he'd just finished shooting in which he not only starred, but also made his directorial debut. This time he was calling the shots, thereby asserting himself in a truly positive and empowering way. Being in charge had allowed him to take back his power from the many directors who had walked all over him in the past.

As Brian told me about making the film, I could feel the change in him. I could see it too. Not only was he more present and confident, but much of his hair had grown back and thickened.

Following our conversation, he gave my gold coin back to me. "Thank you for lending this to me," he said, "but I don't think I'll be needing it anymore."

Brian had come to me thinking he needed help with his thinning hair, whereas what he really needed was help finding clarity by addressing the sense of powerlessness that had intruded upon his professional life. Once he did so, he was able to move his career forward, not to mention feeling better and more fulfilled in every aspect of his life. His body then responded by resuming normal hair growth because, in ways you will come to understand during the course of this book, our biography dictates our biology.

Achieving Clarity

Clarity is the difference between being unable to assert yourself and having a healthy self-image. It's what stands between having a combative relationship with your significant other or a supportive relationship. It's what allows you to go from being the kind of parent who loses it in tricky situations to someone who's capable of soothing, guiding, and modeling positive behavior. It can even be the difference between life and death.

Clarity, in other words, is pivotal.

All this may sound like a bit of magic right now, but I assure you that clarity can make this kind of radical difference in your life. I can also assure you that it's within the grasp of every single person on the planet. If you give it a chance, you'll see for yourself. Part II will take you through a step-by-step process, complete with practices and exercises you can do on your own, that will help you bring greater clarity into your life.

By the end of this process, you will not only know how to create clarity but also how to maintain it over the long term. What we all need moving forward is a clean, unadulterated space inside us—an unbiased, uncluttered context in which to process all the information, emotions, relationships, and events that are still to happen in our lives. We also need to know how to maintain this space by practicing good psycho-spiritual hygiene.

Once you know how to do this, there will be nothing standing in your way as you consciously choose the life you wish to lead. You will no longer stumble over the distractions, prejudices, beliefs, and stored-up energy that most of us have to manage every day *before* we can begin to deal with new situations or make new decisions.

Having clarity doesn't mean having all the answers all the time. Instead it means having a kind of internal GPS so you always know how to figure out what to do and where to go, no matter what you're facing. It means having the psycho-spiritual space you need to process and make sense of every experience that happens in your life, so you know what to take from it and what to leave behind. In this way all of your experiences become an opportunity to learn, grow, and expand your world.

In the next chapter we'll explore some new, empowering ways of looking at the world and at ourselves, which will put you in a more beneficial frame of mind to start your journey toward clarity.

....

"Man longs for certainty, but that he cannot have. We cannot know, and should not try to know, the future of human society. No man has any right to assert: We will come through, or even: A favorable outcome is probable. Probability is irrelevant to history; there exist no measurable factors determining what our fate shall be. We can only know what is possible.

"But if we cannot have certainty we can at least have clarity, the redeeming clarity of the world view of man in nature, years or decades before the sciences give it their indirect confirmation. However, to accept this, man must have been purged of his prejudices such as being in an extreme degree pro or anti science or religion and be prepared for fresh hard thinking, open to the new everywhere. He must use his imagination, blunted as it has been at the deeper levels by technology and industrialism. Moreover, he must accept this fact: Clarity carries no guarantee of any kind, of survival, of success. Clarity is an aesthetic, not a utilitarian value.

"What, then, does the world view imply for man's conception of himself, his feelings, his thoughts, and his actions? This above all: morphic man knows that every life-enhancing impulse in himself is an expression of the organic tendency toward coordination, itself an expression of the universal morphic tendency. This awareness runs through many levels of his mind.

"At one level man experiences freedom of choice; he feels himself to be a free agent seeking order and harmony. But at a deeper level, aware of more, he knows himself to be less than free, the instrument of forces greater than himself. There is no contradiction here. The old antithesis of free will and necessity vanishes in the hierarchical view of man. The 'higher' levels of the mind express more specialized factors, the 'lower' more general. At one level he experiences freedom of choice, but when he becomes aware of the deepest level of all, he loses free will and experiences the bliss of enjoying and serving a pervasive unity. For joy is simply vitality without discord."

—Lancelot Law Whyte, *The Universe of Experience: A Worldview beyond Science and Religion*

CHAPTER TWO

The Need for a Clarity Mindset

Clarity is in short supply in our world today. There are symptoms of this shortage all around us. You see it in our political system, where so many are so certain that they have the "right" answers even when they directly contradict the "right" answers of those across the aisle. You see it in people who find themselves in the same unwanted situations again and again and think it's just bad luck that the pattern keeps recurring in their lives.

Why is it so hard for so many of us to find clarity?

To understand the challenge, we have to realize that we all divide our time between two worlds—the external, made up of the people and things we see all around us, and our own personal internal world, which is unseen and contains our thoughts, feelings, and ideas. For all its benefits, modern society tends to keep us focused on our external reality, causing us to neglect our internal world. It's as if our society supports, even promotes, an oversaturated, overcluttered, overstressed, and hence confused state of being.

A number of forces contribute to this confusion. One is that as our culture has become more secular, we have lost our rituals. This isn't an endorsement of any particular religion or even of religion in general. However, much of religious or spiritual practice tends to direct people to focus on their internal world and connect with their spiritual selves. Through rituals such as confession and fasting (which all major religions seem to have, from Lent to Yom Kippur or Ramadan), people think of themselves as practicing a kind of internal cleansing, a spring-cleaning of the mind and body. As a society we don't engage in these kinds of rituals as often as we used to.

Rituals have long served as forms of internal hygiene, a kind of psycho-spiritual handwashing. We practice the art of cleanliness through regular handwashing, before meals and after using the restroom in order to keep our hands free of dirt and germs even when we can't see the contaminants. In the same way, a regular psycho-spiritual washing keeps our internal world free from the muck that can build up inside it.

What happens when we don't psycho-spiritually wash on a regular basis? Picture your kitchen sink the last time you let it go for a while, or remember the hoarder's home I described previously. Our internal world progresses from cluttered to dirty to just plain unhealthy the longer we ignore or neglect it. Clarity is the antithesis of this.

Living in a technological era is another reason clarity can be elusive. It's no secret that technology is changing the way we think and act, a large part of which is down to the way we've become accustomed to speed and instant gratification. Once upon a time we put a letter in the mail when we wanted to communicate with someone far away, then waited weeks, even months, for a reply. Now we send an email, a text, or a tweet and expect an instant response. We wait impatiently as our microwaves take a minute or two to cook something that would have taken at least ten times as long before this technology became available.

The rushed nature of modern life isn't conducive to clarity. Clarity requires space. It requires that we slow down so we can hold our thoughts and feelings rather than rush past them on to the next thing. The conditions needed for creating clarity are, in essence, the exact opposite of what we've come to expect from living in a fast-paced, instantly gratifying, technological world.

What's more, technology has intensified a trend that was already taking place in our culture, which is an increasing loss of connection and context. There was a time when humans ate only what grew near them. Most communication took place face-to-face. Most learning happened through experience. Now the rice we eat for dinner comes from India while the tomato comes from New Jersey. Professions of love might come not from our partner's lips but through characters appearing suddenly and unexpectedly on a screen. We may have hundreds of "friends" on Facebook or "followers" on Twitter but rarely if ever spend any time with these people in person. We're becoming increasingly *disconnected* from that which feeds us, both physically and spiritually. In other words, so much of what happens in our lives is out of context, whereas clarity both requires and creates context.

Today more than ever the practice of clarity is vitally important. Because so much in our world pushes to obscure relationships and cloud healthy connections, we need something to counteract these effects. We need to start by cultivating a new mindset, which begins when we adopt what I call the Clarity Mindset.

The Clarity Mindset is a set of ideas that usher in a new perspective, a fresh way of thinking and looking at the world that can help us create the psycho-spiritual space we need to better process and make sense of our experiences and bring us the lives we want.

Think of the Clarity Mindset like walking into a room and seeing a light switch that's either on or off. If this is the only kind of light switch we've ever seen, we think those are the only two options available. Imagine then encountering a new kind of switch—a dimmer. Instead of limiting us to on or off, we now have a range of options from no light at all to the brightest setting and everything in between. This is the kind of mindset shift we're aiming for.

To go from an on-off mentality to a dimmer mentality requires a change of consciousness. It means moving from a dualistic point of view where things are either on or off, good or bad, right or wrong, to one where there are varied shades in between. Of course, whereas a basic on-off light switch can cost as little as a dollar, even the cheapest dimmer is typically four times as much since the technology required to make it work is that much more complex and therefore more costly to produce. Nevertheless, the benefits far outweigh the cost.

Just as using a dimmer gives us more options in terms of the light in the room, shifting our consciousness to the Clarity Mindset provides us with the options we need to create the life we want.

Being Stuck Is Unnatural

This diagram shows in simple terms the relationship between our external and internal worlds. The external world, on the left, is where we encounter things that are visible and concrete. It's also where we project our judgments of the things we encounter, such as "I don't like that person" or, "This situation isn't good for me." This is why it's labeled the "judgmental realm." The right side is the internal world, where we encounter the invisible and abstract, like our thoughts, feelings, memories, and ideas. I call this the "imaginal realm," and it's the realm that's most often neglected in our world today.

Getting stuck in the judgmental realm is a common problem. Someone who spends a majority of their time in the judgmental realm will often be highly opinionated and unable to tolerate, let alone integrate, new ideas or differing opinions. This is the situation we see frequently in politics—people whose opinions have become so solidified and so calcified from spending too much time in the concrete world that when they talk about them, they sound like they're

Cycle of Life

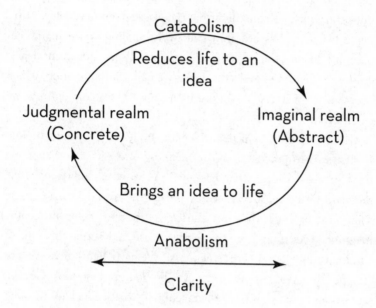

Catabolism

Reduces life to an idea

Judgmental realm (Concrete)

Imaginal realm (Abstract)

Brings an idea to life

Anabolism

Clarity

describing unalterable truths rather than personal beliefs. They also tend to sound like they're stuck on repeat and unable to move on— like an old vinyl record caught in a groove. It's clear just by listening to them that there's no room for movement no matter how someone might respond to what they're saying and regardless of the quality of the other person's opinions.

I don't mean to suggest that the judgmental realm is bad or should be avoided altogether. Remember, we are working toward a dimmer rather than an on-off mentality, which means there's no right or wrong. It isn't my intention to prioritize one side over the other, since life is about both of these worlds. One doesn't exist without the other, and life is best lived when there's a balance between the two.

The new perspective we are working toward is an understanding that the natural world doesn't want us to be stuck in one world or the other. Life depends on movement. Consider how the ocean tides constantly ebb and flow, that the planet itself never stops turning, and our bodies are always at work inhaling and exhaling air, pumping blood, and processing nutrients. When our natural processes are disrupted and slow down, we call it inflammation, which is how disease starts. When our natural processes stop entirely, we call it death.

Clarity allows us to move through the cycles of life uninterrupted. It allows us to process and give meaning to everything. When we don't process things, what happens? As we've already seen, they build up inside us. Everyone recognizes the experience of having some hurt or anger they just can't let go of and seeing it become magnified over time. Even the words we use to describe this type of situation convey a sense of "stuckness." We have "pent-up" anger, are "trapped" in a vicious cycle, or have "bottled up" emotions. Getting stuck is an unnatural state of being, and if we stay stuck for too long it can have a profoundly negative effect on us emotionally, spiritually, and physically. The problem is that when many of us feel stuck, we don't know what to do about it. In fact, we often feel like there's nothing we can do.

Because being stuck is an unnatural state, there's *always* something we can do. Given that both the world and we ourselves are ever changing, we are never stuck, our circumstances are never fixed, and we are never set in our ways.

It will prove extremely helpful to incorporate this realization into your thinking as you move forward. You will be working toward becoming more fluid, more flexible, more able to bend, which will give you more options in life. As Bruce Lee once said, "Be formless, shapeless like water. Now, you put water into a cup, it becomes the cup. Put it into a teapot, it becomes the teapot.... Be water, my friend." Why like water? Because while water can adjust to any situation, it will never break no matter how much pressure you put on it. That's how we are aiming to be, flexible but unbreakable.

Your Body and Mind Are One

This next mindset shift requires us to change our view of *ourselves*. Rather than seeing our body and mind as two separate entities, we want to see them as parts of the same system, the same whole.

It's common for people to talk about their personal problems in physical terms. "He's such a pain in the neck" someone comments. "I just can't shoulder the weight of it any longer" another remarks. Even though we use such expressions, we don't seem to make the connection between the psycho-spiritual and the physical.

There was a time in human history when the link between mind and body *was* well understood, particularly in relation to a person's health. Socrates said, "There is no illness of the body apart from the mind." The term *psychosomatic* comes from the ancient Greek, where *psycho* means mind and *soma* means body. Healers at that time believed all illness was psychosomatic, or a mind-body event, requiring treatment on both fronts. Sadly today we use the term to suggest an illness that's all in your head.

If you really think about it, this modern definition comes from a strange perspective. We are one being, one system, and yet we so often treat the mind and the body as if they were separate entities with some sort of impenetrable wall between them. We go to a different kind of doctor to treat the body than to treat the mind. We often talk about body and mind as if they were in opposition to each other, as seen in the expression "my body says yes but my mind says no." The truth is, the body doesn't function separately from the mind. They are intimately and intrinsically tied together. Since we can't separate one from the other, why when we are suffering do we try to attribute our condition to one at the exclusion of the other?

The reason a shift in our mindset is so important is that without it we can't clearly see the root mindset of our suffering. A common complaint about the way Western medicine is practiced is that physicians treat physical symptoms but far too often fail to address the cause of a condition. My approach is to look not at an isolated set of symptoms but at the total functioning of my patients, mind and body together. I believe the vast majority of disease is psychosomatic. Although it's a condition of the mind *and* the body, 99 percent of the time its origin is in the mind.

When we are unable to process the negative energy that results from unwanted experiences or emotional upset, it can't pass through us. As a result it ends up becoming stuck within us. Research has shown that negative judgments and emotions actually resonate on the cellular level, disrupting our natural biological frequency. Over time this negative energy builds up. Eventually we become completely saturated with it, subconsciously incorporating our resentment, guilt, inadequacy, and so on into our personality. This creates dis*ease* in our consciousness, which if left unchecked erupts as disease in either our bodies or life situation, and sometimes both. Sickness is the end result of a lack of clarity left to fester over time.

This was what I saw with Lisa, a 38-year-old, high-powered attorney who was suffering from debilitating rheumatoid arthritis. A chronic disorder, rheumatoid arthritis is an immune system malfunction in which a person's body begins attacking its own joints. The swelling in Lisa's hands and feet was so bad that it caused her near-constant pain and was interfering with her work. Unable to understand why this condition had appeared in her life at such a young age and seemingly out of the blue, she felt utterly frustrated. She also couldn't understand why the only help she had received from the previous physicians she'd seen was in the form of recurring prescriptions for powerful painkillers that only partially deadened her pain, had unwanted side effects, and did little to alleviate her condition over the long term.

Like many people, Lisa assumed her condition was only physical, so she wasn't looking within herself for contributing factors when she came to see me. Nor were her previous doctors. I got a sense of what might be influencing her disease when I asked her when her symptoms initially appeared. She explained, "I first experienced them while sailing with my husband off the coast of San Diego. It was just a little excursion we took when I went out to visit him. We'd been apart for several months at the time because of his job. He'd been living in Southern California, where he was setting up a new office for his firm. Our daughter and I had stayed behind on the East Coast so she could finish the school year and I could sell the house. The plan was to join him after that."

The sudden onset of Lisa's symptoms after being reunited with her husband piqued my curiosity, so I questioned her further. I wanted to know more about their relationship and what it had been like to be apart for so long. Her resistance to this line of questioning was immediate and obvious. When I didn't let the subject drop, this resistance quickly turned into anger. "What the f*&k does all this have to do with anything?" she finally yelled at me, her face bright red.

Lisa's outsized reaction suggested I had really touched on something, so I stood my ground. "It seems like my questions really triggered you," I told her gently. "I want you to know that I'm here for you and that I want to help you."

I could see the tension building inside Lisa, and I was preparing myself for a brutal retort when, to my surprise, she broke down and started weeping. That was when she told me her story. Almost immediately after her husband left for San Diego, she had begun a passionate affair with a woman in her neighborhood. Although she felt the affair was wrong, she said it was like a drug for her. Despite her intense guilt, she simply couldn't tear herself away. Six months after the start of the affair, she found herself on the romantic sail-boat trip with her husband in San Diego Bay, which triggered the onset of her symptoms.

After further prompting, Lisa revealed that deep down she felt like she deserved the painful disease she was suffering from. It seemed an appropriate punishment for betraying her husband. She felt so badly about what she'd done that her own body was attacking her for it.

When Lisa revealed this to me, although it had been a year since she'd ended the affair, her symptoms hadn't improved at all. She thought arthritis was her only problem, but her persistent illness pointed to something else. It was obvious to me that her body wouldn't stop punishing her until she stopped suppressing her guilt and punishing herself for her actions. The healing she so badly needed would only come when she understood how her emotional state was contributing to her physical illness and did something about it.

It wasn't easy, but Lisa began to heal herself emotionally by owning up to what she'd done, forgiving herself, and giving her husband a chance to do the same by being honest with him. The two of them entered counseling together and over time their marriage began to heal, followed by the healing of her physical symptoms.

Today this couple are still together and profess to be happier than ever. Lisa no longer needs the powerful painkillers she was taking to cope with her arthritis. In fact she takes no medication at all. As she learned to be kinder to herself, letting go of her guilt and self-judgment, her body learned to be kinder to her as well.

Your Reality Is a Projection

The shift we need to make is to move from thinking of our experience of reality as a set of cold, hard, unalterable facts to understanding it as a projection of our inner world. Most of us have no idea why things happen in our lives because we see only what's happening in our outer world. We determine *he/she/it* did this *to me,* or even *I* did this to *myself,* which means *I am* _____ *and I don't/can't/shouldn't/will never* _____ as a result.

In Lisa's case, she might fill in the blanks by saying, *I did this to myself by having an affair, which means I am a terrible person and I don't deserve to be happy.* Someone who has been cheated on might say, *My husband did this to me, which means I'm not worthy of love and will end up alone.*

The conclusions drawn in both of these cases aren't cold hard facts. They come from limiting beliefs those concerned hold about themselves in their inner worlds. Lisa didn't need to forsake love for the rest of her life just because she had an affair, and someone who has been cheated on isn't unworthy of love. Yet punishing beliefs like these have a way of implanting themselves in our subconscious. Once implanted, they drive our behavior.

The reason this happens has to do with how our brains work. The subconscious behaves this way, in part, to try to make life easier for us by bypassing the need to think everything through. For example, when we were first learning to tie our shoes, we had to focus on every step in the process. Today if we knelt down to tie our shoes, our hands would fly through the steps without us having to think about them. It saves us a lot of time and effort to be able to do things like this automatically.

Being on autopilot is great when it comes to things like tying shoes, but it's not so great and can be very damaging if, for example, we were told or shown over and over again in childhood that we didn't deserve love and, as a result, our subconscious integrated this belief and carried it into adulthood. The subconscious doesn't judge the quality of our beliefs. It simply trusts that we are the expert when it comes to knowing what's best for us, then guides us toward people and situations that validate our deepest beliefs.

The problem comes of course when our entrenched beliefs are inaccurate, even detrimental to us, but still lead us to make choices that reaffirm what we believe. This is why so many find themselves repeating the same unwanted patterns, like getting divorced...again, or finding themselves caught in a dead-end job...again. They aren't reacting to the situation in front of them, they are reacting to the history stored in their subconscious.

This might sound like we are doomed to be controlled by the subconscious beliefs that are limiting our lives, but this isn't the case. Life isn't predetermined and we aren't robots running along a preset track. At least, we don't have to be. Once we shift our mindset and understand that our version of reality is shaped by our subconscious beliefs, we can consciously choose to alter our thought processes to trigger new behavior that better serves us.

As we journey toward clarity, consider the idea that, without exception, our perception of everything in our outer world is a projection of some part of our inner reality. While our subconscious thoughts aren't immediately accessible to us (they're subconscious, after all), they make themselves known in our reaction to situations.

An old saying goes, "You spot it, you got it." It means we can't recognize a quality within another person unless we have some element of it in ourselves. To illustrate how this works, at some point in your life you've probably encountered a coworker who irritated you for some reason. The person's behavior got on your nerves, but why didn't it affect everyone else in the office in the same way? Because everyone else didn't have a belief in their subconscious that was triggered by the coworker's behavior.

A movie projector needs a screen on which to project images, otherwise the light just travels away from it and gets lost. In much the same way, your subconscious uses external objects like people and situations as screens on which to project beliefs. So the next time you feel like ranting at someone for disrespecting you, consider the possibility that your subconscious has created the experience to awaken you to the fact that you subconsciously don't respect *yourself*. Why else would you continually put yourself in the company of people who treat you poorly?

Our subconscious uses projections to get our attention and show us what's happening in our internal world. When we fail to understand the messages it's projecting for us, we continue to reinfect ourselves with negative emotional energy. This is when the body starts trying to get our attention in the form of pain or other symptoms.

Projections are simply a form of information, a communication from our internal world, a clue as to what's happening in our subconscious. If we understand this and pay attention, every situation we encounter becomes an opportunity to learn something about ourselves. If what's being projected pleases us, then great. If not, we have a chance to uncover the subconscious belief that supports it and work to release it. By releasing it we make room for more-empowering beliefs to take hold. This is what clarity means. It's also the only way significant change can happen in our lives.

We'll look more closely at how to do this in the next section, but for now what's important to understand is that reality as we generally think of it—as some static, incontrovertible truth—is irrelevant. This is because I will never see the "reality" of an object or an event in the exact same way you will, since everything we experience is filtered through our own individual ways of understanding and interpreting the world. In other words, reality is irrelevant and perception is everything. It's the way we perceive things that we want to have a better, clearer relationship with in order to lead fuller lives.

Our situation reminds me of the story of the princess and the pea. The princess was so sensitive that she could feel one little pea beneath a stack of mattresses. If she could feel that something so small was off in her environment, then she could do something to change it. That takes a high degree of clarity. In our case, the more clarity we have, the more easily we can perceive the peas that are disrupting our world.

I believe that life is a continuous series of experiences designed to increase our understanding of ourselves and our internal and external worlds. The way we react to those experiences isn't predetermined. We have a choice, but only if we pay attention to the messages our internal world sends us—in other words, to our projections.

Many people don't know who they are, so they look outside of themselves for the answer. They measure their worth by how many followers they have on Facebook or Twitter, what sort of title they've been awarded in their career, or how the people around them see and react to them.

Looking outside yourself for the answer to such a profound question as who you really are is a useless endeavor, one that will only cause you to have a skewed view of yourself. Looking outside yourself for why you're experiencing difficulties in your life won't solve your problems either. It will only cause you to re-create the same negative experiences again and again.

In other words, if you don't like the tea you're currently drinking, don't blame the person who served it to you. Instead choose to brew your own tea. Deciding which tea will serve you best starts with listening closely to the messages your inner world is trying to send you.

Seeing Problems as Possibilities

Life has a rhythm. The sun rises as the moon recedes, only to set again, making way for the moon once more. Wildfires burn the forest, but just days later new growth appears. The natural world lies dormant in winter, only to reemerge with new life each spring. Everything is bound by this natural rising and falling pattern. I call it the metabolism of life.

On every level, life is constantly breaking itself down (a process known as catabolism) only to build itself back up again (anabolism). Our bodies follow the same pattern as hundreds of millions of cells die each day and are replaced by new ones. In fact, in just under two years, not a single cell in our current body will still be alive. It's like we all get a brand-new body every couple of years. Contemplate this incredible truth for just a moment. Not a single cell in your current body existed at the time you were born. Yet despite the fact that the physical matter making up your body has been renewed many times over, you are still you.

Most of us recognize this continuous rhythm in nature but fail to understand how it applies to our individual circumstances. As with nature, our lives have catabolic and anabolic phases, or ebbs and flows. When we move from the judgmental to the imaginal realm, that's the catabolic or breaking-down phase. We break down judgments to free the imagination. When we move in the opposite direction, from imaginal to judgmental, that's the anabolic or building-up phase. We move from the abstract to the concrete in order to bring an idea to life. As we've learned, we are at our best when we are constantly moving between the two realms.

Humans are prone to comparing and contrasting things. When we look at a coin, we tend to see it as having two sides. Opinions or behaviors are either right or wrong. People are good or bad. Something either serves us or hurts us. When we view the natural phases of our lives, we tend to consider the happy, opening up, springlike times (the anabolic phase) to be good and the winters of sadness and hardships (the catabolic phase) to be bad. I would like to suggest a new way of looking at things.

Because we can't have spring without winter, and we can't have flow without an ebb, why judge them? If we step back and look at the entire picture, we'll see that both are necessary to move us forward. Just as a ship uses the rise and fall of waves to get to its destination, to navigate through our lives and get where we want to go we must learn to work with all the natural rhythms of life instead of fighting against half of them. A life with no ebb, no winter, no moon simply isn't possible. What's more, it wouldn't be very interesting.

As we move through the process of creating clarity, my hope is that you will begin to shift your thinking in this way. I say this because when we stop defining challenging situations as "bad," we start seeing the possibilities inherent within them—yes, even in our most difficult times and our deepest traumas.

To help my patients understand this, I often ask them to picture an archer stepping up with his or her bow and arrow to shoot at a target. How does the bow work? I've asked this question of numerous patients and most think it's the string that stretches as the archer pulls his or her arm back to shoot. But this isn't the case. It's the bow that changes, bending but not breaking under the pressure applied to it. Imagine what it would be like if we were more like a bow, allowing the pressure of even our greatest challenges to shape us rather than break us.

By adopting this way of thinking, problems big or small no longer need to be avoided, repressed, or even lamented. Instead they can be seen as opportunities for learning, growing, and healing. They are the winters that lead to our psycho-spiritual spring. We can come to see all the events of our lives, especially our problems, as serving our highest good. We might even say there's no such thing as a problem, only an opportunity to create a better life.

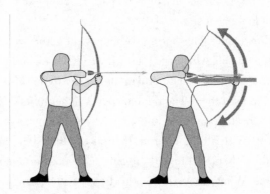

....

KEY MINDSET SHIFTS

....

1. Being stuck is unnatural. Movement is the natural order of things.
2. Body and mind aren't separate, but together make up one whole.
3. Our outer world reflects what's happening in our inner world.
4. Problems are opportunities for growth.

....

"The spirit is the master; imagination the tool, and the body the plastic material. ... The power of the imagination is a great factor in medicine. It may produce diseases in man and in animals, and it may cure them. Ills of the body may be cured by physical remedies or by the power of the spirit acting through the Soul."

—Paracelsus, the Father of Toxicology

ಲ್ಲಿ

THE PROCESS OF CREATING CLARITY

What to Expect from Part II

If all this seems a bit difficult to grasp, don't worry. A true mindset shift takes time and requires a little space. The key thing right now is to simply keep these concepts in mind as you move forward. You'll practice internalizing and manifesting them in Part II as you make your way, step by step, through the process of creating clarity.

And clarity *is* a process, meaning it isn't something you snap your fingers to bring about. So as you make your way through Part II, go slowly. It's okay for progress to be incremental. In fact slow but steady progress should be your goal. After all, it takes far longer to build a skyscraper than it does to bring one down with the wrecking ball, and you are aiming to build something big. You aren't trying to simply change a habit or a particular way of thinking. You are trying to build a whole new process, an entirely new way of being that will last for the rest of your life. Change on this scale happens slowly, so you want to embrace this fact instead of putting pressure on yourself to speed the process along. The process is the goal here. I can give you a quick recipe for making kimchi, but no recipe can tell you what the experience of making it and eating it yourself is like. Remember this as you move from step to step. Take time to savor the process.

Another thing to keep in mind as you make your way through Part II is that you may be asked to do things or think in ways you object to or that make you feel uncomfortable. I have often seen patients latch on to one concept they disagree with and use it as a reason to abandon the whole process.

If you put enough pressure on any object, it will eventually crumble. If what you are looking hardest for are flaws, that's what you'll find. If there are ideas or stories in this book that you take issue with for one reason or another, or things I could have explained more clearly or precisely, try not to let this divert you from your path. In other words don't throw out the baby with the bathwater, as they say. This is especially important because, in my experience, the people who most need clarity are also the ones who most resist it.

One last word of advice. Along the way, be curious! This process is meant to stir you up and poke you in order to reveal your weak points so they can be brought into the light. Acknowledge whatever surfaces, even if you don't yet know what it means or what to do with it. Resist the urge to turn away from discomfort or pain and instead be inquisitive. The more you're willing to ask questions and explore, the more clarity you'll find.

Let's get started!

Take Responsibility for Your Emotional Waste

Not long ago my wife and I decided to look for a new home outside Los Angeles. We've been city dwellers our entire lives, so house hunting outside a metropolitan area was an education for us. Among the things we had to learn was that homes in the country aren't on a municipal sewer system. Instead they each come equipped with a private underground septic system. As I got to know more, I became fascinated with how simple and ingenious these systems are and what they can teach us about processing other kinds of waste in our lives such as emotional waste.

As a physician who works in mind-body medicine, I believe we all need our own private internal system for processing our emotional waste. Yet in the modern world in which we live, many of us feel that processing emotional waste isn't our responsibility. Instead we abdicate the responsibility to external sources. We do this in any number of ways, including blaming others for our problems, succumbing to addiction, or placing the responsibility on a partner, parent, therapist, guru, or member of the clergy to do it for us.

I used to go for psychoanalysis on a regular basis, until one day

I realized something I found upsetting. I was struggling with some feelings, but instead of trying to understand what they meant I found myself putting them on hold until my next appointment with my analyst. I realized then that, after all the time I'd spent working with him, what I'd learned above all else was to rely on *him* when difficult emotions came up. What I hadn't learned was how to handle my feelings myself.

I don't mean to suggest that therapy has no place in people's lives, but I do think that over time it can become a poor substitute for learning how to process our feelings for and by ourselves. I believe it's up to each of us to keep our own emotional house clean and, as odd as it may sound, the septic tank can help us understand how to do just that.

What Septic Systems Can Teach Us about Ourselves

How do septic systems work? Simply put, all drainage pipes inside a rural home or business flow into a single pipe and empty into a 2,000 gallon tank located underground some 30 to 50 feet from the structure being served. The tank has dual chambers and as the contents flow from one chamber to the next, bacteria that occur naturally in the anaerobic environment (meaning an environment free from oxygen or air) work to dissolve the solids. Eventually the resulting liquid ends up about 100 feet away in a leach field. Here a gravel-soil mixture filters out any remaining impurities. At this point, what was once a waste product has been purified enough thanks to the work of the bacteria and natural filters that it becomes useful as the last remnants are taken up by the root systems of plants for hydration and eventual transpiration.

It's amazing to think that nature doesn't need anything special in order to transform and purify our bodily waste, just the natural environment. The same is true of our bodies. All food, even the healthy kind, leaves us with byproducts that need to be eliminated, and our bodies have a highly effective means of handling those byproducts through the process we know as digestion.

Likewise the events of our lives leave behind a waste product in the form of residual negative energy that's unhealthy for us if it sticks around too long. I believe we possess within us everything we require to process this energy, but we have to take responsibility for building the system that allows us to do it effectively. Without a proper means of processing and purging these emotions, they build up inside us. Over time they become toxic and contaminate our relationships and our sense of self. This emotional constipation can even make us physically ill.

If I may be blunt, being an emotional and spiritual adult means taking care of our own shit. If we are ever to be psycho-spiritually independent and cultivate healthy soil for our own souls, we must stop processing our emotional waste through other people. We must cease filtering our blame, anger, resentment, jealousy, and depression through external sources like our parents, spouses, siblings, bosses, children, and anyone else on whom we choose to project our feelings. Of course, this requires taking 100 percent responsibility for our current life condition. Such an independent approach leaves us with no option other than to set up our own emotional waste management system.

Creating Our Own Waste-Processing System

As the saying goes, shit happens. There's no escaping it. Most of the time we interpret this phrase as referring to the big problems that arise in our lives, but small negative situations bombard us every day too and are in fact more dangerous and toxic to us because they occur so frequently. These little assaults on clarity need to be neutralized on a daily basis lest they build up and become yet one more big problem that we imagine "just happened."

Any real estate agent will tell you that a house with a faulty septic system is virtually unsellable. Left abandoned and at the mercy of the elements, it will simply break down into a pile of rubble. Without the ability to fully process and eliminate dangerous emotions, the same happens to us. When we neglect our emotions by avoiding or burying them, we begin to break down mentally and physically. The best guarantee we can provide ourselves for robust health and emotional wellbeing is to build our own internal emotional waste management system and continually care for it so it stays in good working order. This is how we start bringing clarity into our lives.

When my patient Sharon first came to see me, she had practically no way at all of processing her emotions. Of course, this wasn't why she arrived in my office. At the age of 29, this advertising executive was suffering from digestion problems so severe that practically anything she ate was violently rejected by her body. With few exceptions, the simple act of ingesting food led to diarrhea, gas, bloating, and always pain. Dreading another bout of extreme discomfort, she found herself skipping meals on a regular basis, trying instead to nourish herself on liquids and vitamins, the result of which was an unintended but serious loss of weight.

This poor woman had traveled all over the world visiting doctors she hoped could help her, spending nearly her entire life savings in the process. She had been diagnosed with everything from irritable bowel syndrome (IBS) and colitis to Crohn's disease, but sadly none of the remedies prescribed had brought her relief. By the time she arrived in my office she was at her breaking point. In fact the very first thing she said to me was, "I just can't do this anymore."

Based on my tests and observation, I told Sharon I was quite certain she had been misdiagnosed. In my experience, patients who have difficulty digesting food often have trouble digesting emotional experiences as well. This pattern proved to be true for Sharon and dated back to early childhood. She had grown up with a mother who suffered from bipolar disorder and was "all over the place" emotionally. Although Sharon herself wasn't bipolar, as she developed into an adult, she found she exhibited the same inability to contain her emotions as her mother. Her reactions to problems were always more exaggerated than the actual circumstances warranted, leaving her unable to manage the details of her life without feeling completely and utterly overwhelmed.

The special diets and pills Sharon had been prescribed hadn't worked because what she really needed was to learn how to effectively digest her emotions. The word *digestion* comes from *di*, meaning "two," and *gestate*, meaning "to carry"—in other words to carry two things at the same time. When we eat, the body takes in what's in essence a foreign substance. The digestive process that nourishes us and keeps us alive requires we hold these foreign substances inside our bodies while they are broken down so we can absorb the nutrients we need and eliminate the rest. To digest anything properly, the body must do two things: (1) hold the substance inside for the right amount of time and (2) extract all the good things from it while releasing what doesn't serve us.

We digest emotional experiences in much the same way. If something upsetting occurs, we must be able to hold the emotional charge it causes within ourselves long enough to be able to process it. This means allowing our emotions to unfold while *at the same time* thinking through those emotions, understanding that in every negative experience there is vital information that will serve us by helping us learn and grow. We digest the experience by extracting these gifts and leaving the other details (self-judgment and feelings of blame or shame, for example) behind. In essence, digesting an emotional experience requires the ability to feel and think at the same time. To put it another way, it's to think through one's feelings.

If we cannot properly digest our emotions, we tend to react by rejecting the situation outright, often dramatically by blaming others and venting our outrage. This is feeling *without* thinking, and it means we are emotionally uncontained. It also means we lack clarity. Because we've emotionally rejected the experience, neither can we absorb the lesson it has brought us, which in turn stunts our ability to grow in self-awareness.

Usually our mothers teach us how to contain our emotions and break them down starting when we are babies, which is why this process can also be called *self-parenting*. One of the main things we aim for as we reach for greater clarity is the ability to self-parent in any situation, which allows us to solve the problems we are presented with rather than (1) expecting someone else to solve them as we adopt a powerless attitude, (2) blaming someone else for them as we adopt an aggressive attitude, or (3) avoiding them altogether by adopting a passive attitude.

When we self-parent, we see and accept a situation as it exists, and then work with it to achieve a positive outcome, learning what we can from the experience along the way. This doesn't mean we have to be happy about what's happening to us or that we allow others to avoid responsibility for their part. If someone commits a crime, we still have them prosecuted. If we're in a damaging relationship, we still get out of it. While we are doing these things, we want to take control of how we process and respond to the experience, taking from it what we can use to move us forward and discarding anything that might keep us stuck.

Because of her disorder, Sharon's mother was unable to teach her how to self-parent properly. That's why, even as an adult, Sharon treated every incident, no matter how small, in the powerless way a child might—as if it were the end of the world. Since there was no one in her childhood to help her break her problems down and assure her everything was going to be okay in the end, she was unable to do these things for herself in adulthood. With no one to model emotional containment for her, she saw the world as a dangerous place and her life as a series of crises, one after another.

Because Sharon couldn't digest her emotional life properly, negative emotional energy built up and was stored within her body, which in time reacted by echoing this dysfunction through her inability to digest food. I'll never forget the look on her face as I explained this to her. By the time I'd finished, she was holding her head in her hands. She finally looked up at me and said, "No one ever told me this."

None of us likes the way problems make us feel, which is why we reject them through blame or denial. However, rejecting problems doesn't make them disappear. I told Sharon it was never too late to let problems in, holding them as she broke them down for her benefit. This is how we avoid getting stuck in our own waste.

To Sharon's enormous credit, after just a few months of following the steps described in this book she was able to process a much wider range of emotions without feeling her world was crumbling. Happily she was also able to digest a much wider range of food without pain or discomfort. She's now able to eat many of her favorite foods again and is back to her original weight. What's more, she continues to learn how to be a loving and protective mother to herself as she takes the last few steps toward full recovery.

WHAT WE CLEAR THROUGH OUR PERSONAL SEPTIC SYSTEM

Our internal emotional waste management system flushes out the things that build up inside us and keep us from finding clarity—the emotions and feelings that keep us from living lives full of happiness, fulfillment, and love:

- emotional residue
- preconceived judgments
- limiting beliefs
- misperceptions about ourselves and our lives
- misperceptions about others and the world around us

Proceed with Intention

When something upsets us, all our attention tends to get directed toward what we believe to be wrong with the situation. However, because energy flows where attention goes, focusing constantly on what we don't want can only bring us *more* of what we don't want.

The first step toward taking responsibility for your emotional waste is to focus your energy where you want it to go by setting a *clear, positive* intention. This will begin building an emotional waste management system that will bring you greater clarity.

By articulating a clear, positive intention that accurately describes how you'd like to see something unfold and eventually find resolution, you shift your focus onto what you *do* want rather than what you don't. For instance, if you want more intimacy in your relationship, you won't find it by focusing on all the ways your partner doesn't provide it. But if instead you set a positive intention to be more open to the ways in which you can create intimacy with your partner, you're much more likely to have the experiences you want.

In a situation involving any kind of relationship, set the intention of building an emotional waste management system to help you proceed with the process of creating greater clarity with regard to improving your relationship with *yourself.* Do it with the intention of finding spiritual fulfillment or healing from trauma. This will improve your relationships with others for the rest of your life.

There's no "right" intention to have, but you do need to set one that feels meaningful to you and serves a positive purpose.

Use the following exercise anytime you want to create a clear, positive intention. Set the intention to build your own emotional waste management system so that you can effectively process your emotions and lead a more positive, peaceful, healthy, and fulfilling life overall—or whatever intention feels right to you.

EXERCISE:
Set Your Intention

Setting a clear, positive intention

- helps you clarify your true desire
- provides a positive goal on which to focus your attention
- reminds you to make positive choices that support your true desire
- gives you the opportunity to access your authentic self to support your highest good.

Your clear, positive intention should be

- uplifting, in the present tense, and relatively broad
- for the highest good of all concerned, including everyone who may be upsetting you
- held in mind, but without rigid attachment. (Don't worry about how your intention will come to pass, just stay open to the possibilities so that you can give the universe unlimited latitude to manifest your intention in the very best way.)
- simple and clear so that it's easy to remember.

DIRECTIONS FOR SETTING YOUR INTENTION

Begin by Calling in Your Authentic Self

Your authentic self is who you really are after all your titles and responsibilities are stripped away. I believe your true identity is the eternal, divine being traveling through this human experience you call your life. Your authentic self exists at a level of consciousness far beyond your present awareness and is sometimes referred to as the Higher Self because it has a bird's-eye view of your entire life experience. Since this authentic self holds an immense amount of information concerning every detail of your life, by becoming conscious of and creating a dialogue with your authentic self you can avoid unnecessary conflict, resolve issues, and find solutions with ease and grace.

1. As you sit in a comfortable position in a quiet place, have a notepad and pen or pencil by your side.
2. Close your eyes and take three deep cleansing breaths. With each exhale, feel more tension leave your body. On the last exhale remain present in the silence for a few moments.
3. When you feel centered, respectfully request (either out loud or internally) that your authentic self be present. Remain still. You may experience a slight shift in your state of being, a subtle calmness that washes over you, or a gentle positivity that lifts your mood. Pay attention to the sensations in your body after making the request. Don't worry if you can't perceive a physical change. Be assured the shift is happening. The authentic self doesn't arrive with emotional fireworks.
4. Sit with this experience for a minute or two, allowing yourself to become acquainted with the quality of its presence. As you

get better at connecting to your authentic self, you'll come to recognize it by its loving presence and a sensation of emotional surrender.

Now Proceed with Creating Your Clear, Positive Intention

1. With your eyes still closed, say either internally or out loud, "Infinite wisdom, I ask for your guidance in *co-creating* the best clear, positive intention for *building my own emotional waste management system* [or whatever issue you are focusing on] that will result in the highest good for myself and everyone involved." Any similar wording will do.

2. Open your eyes, pick up your pen, and start writing whatever comes to mind. Remember, you're embodying your unconditionally loving authentic self right now. It will never judge you, so let go, trust, and allow it to expand within you. Everything you write will ultimately lead you to create your ideal, clear, positive intention.

3. If you find your judgmental self focusing on what you don't want, connect with your authentic self and redirect your thoughts to what you do want.

4. To bring your energy into alignment with your clear, positive intention, express gratitude for the guidance you received and the intention you co-created with your authentic self. You may express your gratitude by writing it out or placing your hand over your heart and allowing feelings of gratitude to flow through you. Any action that has meaning for you will work.

5. Write out your intention on several separate pieces of paper. Handwritten is best, rather than typed on your computer or

phone, for reasons that we will discuss later. Post them in different places around your house and office where you'll see them daily. Carry a copy in your purse or wallet until you've memorized it. It will be your mantra and will help you always stay focused on what you want.

....

EXAMPLES OF CLEARLY EXPRESSED POSITIVE INTENTIONS

....

You are currently using this exercise for the specific purpose of taking responsibility for your emotional waste. However, it can be used anytime you need help focusing your energy in a clear, positive direction. Examples of other intentions you might set as a result of this exercise include the following:

- It's my intention to use my marriage as a tool for my own growth and to always communicate openly and respectfully with my husband/wife.
- It's my intention to set boundaries with my mother and to choose words and actions that strengthen and honor our relationship.
- It's my intention to listen with openness and demonstrate compassion and unconditional love while communicating with my daughter.

....

Acceptance Is Key

The intention you set in the previous exercise will help guide you as you make your way toward greater clarity. As you do this, you will encounter much less resistance on your journey if you practice acceptance. This means trusting the process that has been laid out for you without trying to control it or needing to see the payoff immediately.

Not long ago my wife, Sherry, took me to dinner to celebrate my 20th anniversary of being cancer-free. When we arrived at the restaurant it was obvious this would be no ordinary meal. As we walked in, we were asked to remove our watches and turn off our phones. Sherry placed her hand on the shoulder of our waiter, Michael, and I was prompted to do the same with her. We were then led into a windowless room that was pitch-dark. I soon learned that the restaurant, called Opaque, is run by a staff that's blind.

Unable to see my surroundings, I couldn't orient myself and nearly had a panic attack. But Michael expertly guided us to our table, seated us, and explained how the meal would proceed. Everything had been choreographed and he assured us we were in good hands. As I allowed myself to embrace the situation, something amazing happened. My other senses automatically heightened. The food set before us smelled more vibrant and tasted much richer than anything I had experienced before. My tactile senses were even sharpened as I reached across the table to find Sherry's hand. What started out as disorienting and frightening ended up as an extraordinary, illuminating experience I will never forget.

I would like you to keep this in mind as you take the next steps. An important part of taking responsibility for something is accepting your present circumstances as they are, and then proceeding from there. If you are to take responsibility for your emotional waste, you have to start by accepting that it exists rather than turning away from your negative feelings or pretending they don't exist.

Chances are you found your way to this book because something doesn't feel quite right in your life or because you feel you are somehow in the dark just like I was during that dinner. You might be struggling in a relationship, in need of physical or spiritual healing, or sensing there ought to be more to your life but not knowing how to make it better. The intention you set was likely about finding a positive resolution to this struggle. Whatever your circumstances, no matter how difficult, start by simply accepting what is. Only when we accept our situation can we begin to acclimate to the darkness, then transform our experience into something illuminating and extraordinary.

Cleanse the Body

You have likely heard of, if not participated in, a cleanse, but you probably thought of it as a way to lose weight or improve your physical health. This cleanse is likely to have the same effects, although its purpose is quite different.

You may wonder why we are beginning building an emotional waste management system by focusing on the physical body. The reason goes back to emotions leaving an imprint or residue that gets stored in the body if we don't process them properly. The purpose of this cleanse is to remove the effects of negative energy from your physical body. By doing this early in the process of creating your emotional waste management system, it will prepare your biological terrain for the work to come.

To understand biological terrain, think about the body as a plot of land where you want to grow a beautiful garden. The success of your efforts depends on a lot of variables. What's the quality of the soil? Is it rich with minerals or dry and rocky? If it's the latter, the seeds you plant may not respond. Is the nitrogen level in the soil high or low? The answer to this will affect what will thrive in that particular soil. Are you planting the right seeds for this particular climate? What was the land used for before it came to you? Was it green pasture or a trash heap?

Will the landscaping you've planned affect the irrigation and water runoff? The point here is that every defining factor and decision made about the property in the past and present affect how it performs today.

Another way to think about the past influencing the present is that the body draws on a flowing river of tens of thousands of interconnected and moving parts that come together in a complex choreographed dance. Whatever is introduced to the body upstream in our youth, whether it's a surgery, drug habit, smoking, or sports injury, will intrude upon and change the functional terrain of the body downstream and be felt later in life. As I've said before, our biography dictates our biology.

Because of the link between our minds and bodies, if one is clogged or unwell, so is the other. Remember what Socrates said: "There is no illness of the body apart from the mind." The vast majority of disease has its origin in the mind, which generates our thoughts, which in turn give rise to our emotions, which then resonate at the cellular level.

These two aspects of us, our body and mind, are constantly interacting and impossible to separate. It's therefore important we treat our physical and emotional selves as parts of the same whole, which is why we are cleansing both—first the body in this step, then the mind in the one that follows. We work on cleaning our own terrain in these early steps of our journey so that our soil is ready for the new seeds of clarity we wish to plant.

The Science behind the Cleanse

To cleanse your body, you will spend five days on an eating plan that I call the Intentional Unsaturation Diet, or IU Diet. The IU Diet is designed to remove the physical residue of repressed negative emotions by cleansing and reducing congestion in the organs that are most affected by feelings like resentment and anger. These include the liver, gallbladder, lungs, kidneys, and pancreas.

The IU Diet is what's known as a monodiet. Monodiets involve consuming a large amount of a single or limited number of foods in order to provide the body with a therapeutically significant amount of whole nutrients. The foods that will be ingested in high quantities during this diet are sardines, brown rice, and apples. These foods have been chosen because of their following properties:

- **Sardines:** Most people don't realize that these little fish offer the most complete nutrition per ounce of any food available. They also contain a high dose of B12, a vitamin that supports neural plasticity or the capacity of the nervous system to regenerate and reorganize in response to learning new information, having new experiences, or following an injury. Because we're working on rewiring the brain to view and do things in new ways, neural plasticity is important. It can help us embrace the Clarity Mindset.

- **Brown rice:** Like sardines, this common grain offers a high dose of B12, as well as other B vitamins and minerals the body needs. Just as important, brown rice is the easiest to digest of all the whole grains and has the lowest glycemic index (so you don't get that "peaked blood sugar" effect). Because our intention is to clear out the body, easy-to-process foods are an important component, which is why I recommend eating at least a cup or two of brown rice each day of the cleanse.

- **Apples:** All red fruits—like apples, cherries, and strawberries—have a sugar content made up almost entirely of fructose as opposed to glucose. This is important because fructose doesn't need insulin to enter cells, whereas glucose does. As a result red apples are easier on the pancreas and easier to digest overall.

During this cleanse, I recommend eating apples only after slicing or grating them and leaving them to brown for a while in the open air. When apples have browned, this means they've oxidized, a process that helps break down sugar. All fruits have sugar, but if the sugar has already broken down before you eat it, your pancreas doesn't need to produce insulin to absorb it. Eating red or pink apples (not green ones) that have oxidized (the darker brown the better) is a great way to get some fruit in your diet while also giving your pancreas a break.

By eating these foods, you'll avoid eating other foods that are difficult for your digestive organs to process, causing them to work overtime. Many foods like dairy and sugar tend to be present in high doses in the modern-day diet. This leads to insulin resistance, blood sugar irregularities, and in extreme cases even pancreatic burnout or diabetes. By avoiding certain foods, the IU Diet gives your body a vacation. It lowers your blood sugar, reduces inflammation, and thins out your bodily fluids so they flow more easily. This is a good way to think about the entire process of gaining clarity. Your aim is for things to flow more easily in your life. Remember, one of the mindset shifts we discussed in chapter 2 was that we want things to continually ebb and flow, so anything we can do to increase fluidity in the way we think, the way we process our emotions, or the way our bodies work will result in increased clarity.

THE ROLES OF APPLES AND SARDINES IN THE IU DIET*

	Nutritional Ingredients	Nutritional Benefits
Apples	General	Reduce cancer, cardiovascular disease, asthma, diabetes risk, and cholesterol
	Polyphenolic components Quercetin Bioflavonoids	Antioxidant, anti-inflammatory, hormone-balancing (helps correct estrogen dominance)

*Table and IU Diet derived from *The Theory of Endobiogeny: Volume 1: Global Systems Thinking and Biological Modeling for Clinical Medicine*, Kamyar M. Hedayat, MD, and Jean-Claude Lapraz, MD, Academic Press, 2019.

	Macronutrients Water	Energy, tissue hydration
	Soluble (pectin) and insoluble Fiber	Detoxifies (by absorption and increased evacuation of stool), reduces gallbladder stress, reduces cholesterol and triglycerides, increases HDL (good cholesterol), reduces risk of cardiovascular disease and cancer, helps to maintain healthy body weight
Sardines	Purine proteins	Supports cellular reconstruction, enzymatic function, DNA repair
	Calcium (from chewable bones) Vitamin D	Support bone health, nerve and muscle function, regulation of cellular activity
	Vitamin B12	Supports cardiovascular health
	Omega-3 fatty acids (one of the most concentrated sources)	Anti-inflammatory; reduce cholesterol and triglycerides; reduce risk of heart disease, cancer, and arthritis; support fluidity and integrity of cell membranes; building blocks for hormones
Brown Rice	General	Digests slowly to keep blood sugar levels stable, reduces risk of type 2 diabetes
	Phytonutrients Lignans Antioxidants	Help protect against cancer and heart disease, help protect from free radical damage
	Minerals (trace and major) Manganese Selenium Magnesium	Energy, help protect from free radical damage, reduce cancer and diabetes risk
	Fiber	Detoxifies; reduces gallbladder stress, cholesterol, risk of cardiovascular disease and cancer; helps to maintain healthy body weight

Preparing for the IU Diet

You will derive more from the IU Diet if you prepare yourself and have a good understanding of what you will be doing and why. The tips and ideas that follow will help you get ready and also make the experience easier and more enjoyable.

Go Caffeine-Free

For the duration of this diet, you will be avoiding caffeine entirely because it decreases the effectiveness of our digestive enzymes, making it harder for us to cleanse our system. Food and beverages that contain caffeine also tend to contain high amounts of toxins like pesticides and fungicides, which means they introduce more substances that our bodies need to clear. Additionally, caffeine depletes the amount of growth hormone and creates adrenal fatigue and inflammation, which is the opposite of what we want from an "unsaturation" diet. So avoid coffee, tea (except for caffeine-free herbal varieties), soda, chocolate, or other caffeine-containing items during the cleanse. If you're someone who is used to starting the day with a cup of coffee (or three), then you probably have a caffeine addiction. This is nothing to worry about, although it does mean you'll need to take some extra steps to prepare for the IU Diet so you don't end up with a five-day headache.

Begin by taking stock of how much caffeine you consume in a typical day. You may be well aware of your morning coffee habit, but what about later in the day? Do you drink soda for lunch? Do you often make an afternoon Starbucks run or meet colleagues in the break room for tea or coffee? Before you can wean yourself off caffeine, you'll need to have a good idea of your total daily intake.

Next, reduce your daily caffeine intake by 25 percent. You can do this in any way that works for you. Drink three-quarters of a cup of coffee each time you would typically have a full one or cut out your afternoon coffee break entirely. You may also want to have a substitute on hand. If you drink four cups of coffee each morning, have three cups and a glass of water or juice instead of the fourth cup.

Do this for a few days until your body has adjusted, meaning you aren't feeling sluggish or getting headaches. Then reduce your daily intake by another 25 percent so you're at 50 percent of your original intake.

Continue in this way, reducing gradually, until you're down to zero. This could take anywhere from three to seven days, depending on the amount of caffeine you're used to consuming. Once you've been off caffeine and feeling good for a day or two, you'll be ready to start the IU Diet.

Plan Your Meals and Clear Your Calendar

Take a look at the lists of permitted, emphasized, and restricted foods in what follows to get an overall view of what you'll be eating for the next five days. You may have to change your shopping list for the week, emphasizing fruit and vegetables, while de-emphasizing grains and meat. Also make sure to have plenty of sardines, red or pink apples, and brown rice on hand.

Check your calendar before starting the cleanse to make sure you have five days clear of any events or outings that will make it hard to stick to the diet—a party, for example, where you will want to drink alcohol or a brunch buffet where carbs and desserts will be among the main offerings. If you're unsure what sort of meals to make with the permitted foods, there's a wonderful selection of recipes in the appendix. The recipes are from the test kitchen at Gwyneth Paltrow's lifestyle site, goop (goop.com), and are sure to provide lots of culinary inspiration to help you determine how to plan a variety of meals or use sardines in ways you hadn't thought of before.

Make Plenty of Lemon Water

Every morning when you wake up over the course of your cleanse, you'll drink a large glass of water with lemon (see recipe that follows). Water, of course, is hydrating and will help flush your system. Lemon juice contains vitamin C, citric acid, flavonoids, trace minerals, and other phytonutrients. It also contains antioxidants, has antimicrobial properties, helps eliminate toxins, improves digestion, can treat kidney stones, and supports the immune system. There's even research that suggests the citrus flavonoids in lemons can help prevent and control cancer. Taken together, lemon and water will help you alkalize your body and start your day off right. You can also drink lemon water throughout the day, so make sure to have plenty on hand.

LEMON WATER RECIPE

Use 1–2 whole fresh lemons per liter of water.

1. Wash the lemons, remove any stickers, then chop.
2. Add chopped lemons to a pot of boiling water. Cover and boil for 5 minutes.
3. Remove from heat and steep for 15 minutes more.
4. Strain and drink throughout the day. As an alternative, you can add herbal teas such as chamomile or peppermint to the boiling water.

Eat Breakfast Like a King

There's an old saying that goes, "Eat breakfast like a king, lunch like a prince, and dinner like a beggar." Another version suggests, "Eat breakfast like a lion, lunch like a cat, and dinner like a mouse." Whether you prefer to be a king or a lion, the message is the same. Eat your largest meal early, then consume progressively less throughout the day.

Eating this way will make processing your daily intake of food easier on your body, and the IU Diet aims to be as easy on the body as possible. It will also help you sleep better, which aids digestion and is important for clarity (after all, a groggy mind isn't a clear mind). Research backs up the idea that eating this way benefits our health in a myriad of ways. For example, in *The Blue Zones Solution*, author Dan Buettner takes a close look at the so-called Blue Zones—five regions in Europe, Latin America, Asia, and the United States—that researchers have identified as having the world's highest concentrations of people over the age of 100, and how people who live in these areas eat, including what they eat, how much, how often, and at what times during the day. Among the findings were that people in Blue Zones tend to eat their smallest meal at the end of the day.

When you look at the list of permitted foods, you may think, "Wait a minute, there are hardly any breakfast foods on this list, so how am I going to be able to eat a large breakfast?" If your first meal of the day tends to be loaded with carbs such as cereal, oatmeal, pancakes, muffins, or toast, then this is going to be an adjustment for you. Once again, I ask you to be curious and keep an open mind. For example, when I'm on the IU Diet, I eat sardines and brown rice for breakfast. If the idea of fish for breakfast causes you to recoil, stop for a moment and consider why. After all, lots of cultures have fish for breakfast. Your body surely won't shut down if you eat fish, so why not? What's standing in your way? During the course of this book, you'll be continually encouraged to work to disrupt thought patterns (or what I call holding patterns) that limit you, so fish for breakfast might be a chance to create a new perspective about what breakfast should be. If you can't stomach the idea of sardines in the morning, then try something more familiar. The porridge recipe in the appendix from the goop test kitchen, paired with some fruit, might be a more comfortable option for you.

Half-Day Fasting

The way many of us live today has a disruptive effect on the body's natural rhythms and processes. Eating the largest meal at dinnertime and continuing to eat even after dinner is done, sometimes even snacking late into the night, upsets the body's balance.

During the night, the body goes through a catabolic process, breaking down food, cleansing, and clearing. Our bodies are so active at night that we actually burn more calories in bed than we do when we're awake. By eating large meals late in the day and continuing to eat late at night, we make our bodies work even harder when they're trying to clear. This is often the reason we wake up groggy, stuffy, and in a brain fog. Our bodies are still working to process the previous night's calories. What we want is for the body to have enough time to finish a full cycle of clearing and repair before we start a new day.

In addition to eating a small meal at dinner, we want to let our bodies rest for a full twelve hours during each day of this diet. This means you should plan for twelve hours during which you eat whenever you're hungry, and twelve hours when you don't eat at all. If you plan to eat breakfast at 7:00 a.m., stop eating at 7:00 p.m. the night before. Consider this as a type of mini fast. By fasting overnight, you support the body's natural processes and give it ample time to complete the cleansing process.

Eat Fermented Foods

Because the purpose of the IU Diet is to clear your physical terrain, it's a good idea to think about what you want to reintroduce into the space you will be creating. Fermented foods like kimchi, sauerkraut, miso, tempeh, kefir, and kombucha are great to include in your daily meals during and after the diet to help sustain the effects. These foods contain communities of healthy bacteria that play a role in regulating hormone levels, boosting metabolism, and even increasing the body's uptake of certain vitamins and other essential nutrients. This is why, as you prepare your lunch of brown rice and sardines, you should consider adding a little kimchi on the side.

The Plan: The Five-Day Intentional Unsaturation Diet (IU Diet)

Permitted Foods

Meat (except for day three): poultry, fish, shellfish, and egg whites are okay; all other meats prohibited
Vegetables: no restrictions
Fruit: all fresh varieties, no dried

Emphasized Foods

Apples: only pink or red, sliced or grated and allowed to brown in
the open air
Sardines: fresh or canned in olive oil (smoked are okay)
Brown rice: one to two cups daily
Lemon water: each morning and throughout the day
Fermented foods such as kimchi, sauerkraut, miso, tempeh,
kefir, kombucha, and rejuvelac

Foods to Avoid

Sweeteners of any kind
All nuts and nut products
All grains except for brown rice
Egg yolks
Dairy
Vinegar
Mustard
Legumes (including soybeans and soy products)
Dried fruit
All oils except olive oil
Caffeine
Alcohol

Things to Remember

- Cheating ruins the effects of the diet.
- There are no quantity restrictions, so eat until you're full. In
  particular, eat as many sardines and apples as desired.

- Brown rice is permitted in quantities of one to two cups per day.
- Apples should be eaten only when they turn brown from being exposed to air. Grate or slice them and leave them to brown for as long as possible.
- Apples should be eaten 30 minutes before sardines or three hours after. The reason for eating them 30 minutes before is that the browned apples will help aid your digestion. Sardines and brown rice take about three hours to digest fully, which is why you wait that long afterward to eat more apples. We are aiming to avoid backups and clogs, so this timing is optimal for keeping things moving through your system.
- You can use the following in moderation to dress your food: lemon, fresh or dried herbs, salt and pepper, Bragg Liquid Aminos, ginger, garlic, scallions, onion.

Prescription

Days one to two: eat any foods from all categories, making sure to eat some apples and sardines each day.

Day three: don't eat any meat except sardines.

Days four to five: eat any foods from all categories, making sure to eat some apples and sardines each day.

Note: on each day of the diet, remember to start the day with a large glass of lemon water and to fast overnight for at least twelve hours.

WHAT'S WRONG WITH LEGUMES?

A legume is a vegetable in the pea family. Many people eat legumes as part of a healthy diet, which is fine, just not during this cleanse. We avoid them on this plan because digesting them affects the thyroid and activates the pancreas, creating mucus and thereby increasing viscosity in the body—the opposite of the kind of fluidity we strive for in order gain clarity. Common legumes include all types of beans, peas, lentils, and soybeans.

....

What to Expect from the IU Diet

You will be able to feel the effects of the IU Diet in just a few days. People who have completed the cleanse report having less bloating, less constipation, clearer skin, and more energy overall. I've also measured in my patients a boost in their levels of oxytocin, which is sometimes referred to as one of the "happy hormones" along with serotonin, dopamine, and endorphins. Because of this, you may also experience elevation of your mood during and after the diet. Beyond that, there can be some even more surprising effects.

One of my patients, a woman in her late forties, had been having difficulty getting pregnant for quite some time. She'd had IVF treatments for her first two children, but her third, which came along after she'd completed the IU Diet, was conceived naturally. She and her husband called it a miracle when it happened, but it was likely because the diet affects the body's fluids. Cervical mucus, which is the fluid secreted by the cervix, plays a crucial role in the process of conceiving a child. The amount and quality of a woman's cervical mucus (it can't be too thin or too thick) is important because the fluid helps sperm make its long journey to the place where it can finally fertilize an egg. Because the IU Diet thins out the body's fluids and reduces inflammation, it can quite literally make room for pregnancy. If you have allergies or chronic nasal congestion, you may experience relief from these symptoms during and after the diet for this same reason—a thinning of nasal mucus and a reduction in inflammation.

A patient who had been an insomniac for most of his adult life called me up crying toward the end of his cleanse. For the first time in his life he'd been able to sleep straight through the night. He couldn't believe it and couldn't remember a time when he'd felt so rested.

Another benefit of the cleanse is that it helps balance hormone levels. As I mentioned, I've noticed elevation of patients' oxytocin levels following their completion of the diet, and oxytocin has been shown to modulate the amount of melatonin in the body. Anyone who has ever encountered chronic sleep problems has likely heard about melatonin and the important role it plays in helping our bodies regulate our sleep cycles.

The benefits of this eating plan can be remarkable. However, as you embark on it, you may also find yourself experiencing resistance. You may think you don't like certain foods that are emphasized, such as sardines, or define yourself as a vegetarian or vegan and therefore unable to eat them. If you find yourself in this situation, I'd like to suggest you try to put aside these thoughts and attempt the cleanse anyway.

As mentioned earlier, this diet, and the clarity process in general, asks you to stretch yourself, so if you find yourself saying, "I can't," ask yourself, "Why not?" After all, if you are vegan, I don't think it's likely that eating sardines for a few days is going to kill you or turn you into a "bad" person. I would challenge you to ask yourself what would happen if you prioritized your clarity over your veganism for just a few days. Would that be acceptable? If not, why not? Limiting beliefs can show up in surprising places, even in what we allow ourselves to eat, and we always want to keep in mind that this process is about creating new perspectives and habits that will last us the rest of our lives.

If you find you can only do the first few days of the diet, then start there and proceed from where you are. As you make your way through the steps to come, you will be gaining more and more clarity along the way, so you may find it easier at a later stage to release some of your judgments about what you can and can't eat, what sort of diet you can and can't follow. We will also be revisiting this cleanse in a more advanced form in step eleven of this process, so you'll have another opportunity to try it. Don't beat yourself up about it, but also resist the urge to use a moment of resistance as a reason to abandon your course entirely. You'll likely find yourself uncovering all sorts of similar feelings along the way. After all, unearthing difficult emotions is an integral part of the process, so let's start learning to embrace these moments.

Cleanse the Mind

Kristin was in her late forties when she took up Kundalini yoga. Loving how it made her feel, she started going to classes almost every day. Her experience was dampened however when she started to have painful herpetic outbreaks. During a sexual assault many years earlier, she had contracted genital herpes, a virus that would be with her for the rest of her life but that had typically been dormant ever since. She couldn't understand why these sores were unexpectedly erupting with such force.

That's what prompted Kristin to come to my office for help. When she told me how she had contracted herpes, I asked her to tell me more about the experience. It was so difficult for her to talk about it, she could hardly breathe through most of the retelling. At one point she had to stop talking long enough to vomit.

We came to understand together that, by engaging in so much yoga, she had started to cleanse her physical body and unblock clogged energy. Yoga can be an effective way of achieving this. The problem for Kristin was that she didn't have any way of cleansing her psycho-spiritual self at the same time. She had a lot of repressed emotion that lingered from the traumatic experience, which manifested as physical symptoms that she couldn't ignore.

Kristin's story is a good example of why it's important to cleanse both body *and* mind. Just as our biological terrain is affected by all the things our bodies experience, past and present, so is our psycho-spiritual terrain. The upstream experience of Kristin's assault was being felt downstream in the present day. She had harbored so many negative feelings, including hatred of her own body, blaming herself for what happened, and embarrassment about what her family had been put through because of her experience.

Kristin had a long road ahead of her to process such a difficult experience, the effects of which she had kept buried for many years. But she came to see her herpes outbreaks as a kind of messenger, a clue that her biological and psycho-spiritual terrains were out of balance. With this knowledge, she felt empowered to do something that would help her heal. Cleansing body and mind isn't a cure-all, especially in such extreme circumstances, but it was a starting place that felt manageable. Just as I'm inviting you to do, she started her treatment with the IU Diet and the mind-cleansing exercise that follows later in this step.

I have prescribed this exercise, which I call Purge Emotional Writing, to thousands of patients over the past dozen or so years. It's a basic tool I use in healing because writing is such a powerful mechanism for accessing our innermost thoughts and feelings. This particular exercise uses writing specifically as a cleansing ritual to help detoxify our emotional body of negative energy, in much the same way that the IU Diet cleanses our physical body of negative energy. If you have completed your five-day physical cleanse, it's time to focus on your mind.

We all need ways to help us access our emotions and empty them from our cup. We need to move emotional byproducts through our emotional waste management systems. And the approach we use needs to work on a regular basis. That's what this and the previous step, taken together, are all about. They lay the foundation for clarity by helping us establish rituals for dumping, eliminating, releasing, and clearing space, which are the regular habits of good psycho-spiritual hygiene.

Things come up in our lives all the time. We lose a job. Our friend rejects us or our partner leaves us. Or, more simply, we get stuck in traffic, have an argument with our son or daughter, are overwhelmed at work, or feel stressed when we look at our jam-packed calendar. Any number of situations can call up negative emotions on a daily basis. Purge Emotional Writing, or PEW 12 as I often refer to it (the 12 stands for the twelve-minute time period you will give yourself to write), is an easy way to start processing your emotional waste. It's also an effective ritual to return to anytime your psycho-spiritual terrain is becoming clogged.

The Power of Words

Words have tremendous power, and whether their effects are positive or negative depends on how we choose to use them. I can't express how powerful a tool free-form writing is to expel negative energy from our minds and hearts. I used it daily during my recovery from cancer. I also return to it whenever I'm feeling emotionally oversaturated. No matter what's happening in our lives or what condition we suffer from, I firmly believe in the transformative power of writing to heal us from the inside out.

I'm not the only one who believes this. It's one of the reasons people have kept diaries and journals for generations. There's also ample scientific research to back up the idea. As psychologist Karen Baikie and psychiatrist Kay Wilhelm wrote in their article "Emotional and Physical Health Benefits of Expressive Writing" (*Advances in Psychiatric Treatment*, August 2005),

> Over the past 20 years, a growing body of literature has demonstrated the beneficial effects that writing about traumatic or stressful events has on physical and emotional health.... The immediate impact of expressive writing is usually a short-term increase in distress, negative mood and physical symptoms, and a decrease in positive mood compared with controls. Expressive writing participants also rate their writing as significantly more personal, meaningful and emotional. However, at longer-term follow-up, many studies have continued to find evidence of health benefits in terms of objectively assessed outcomes, self-reported physical health outcomes and self-reported emotional health outcomes.

Those kinds of benefits to our physical and emotional health are what we're aiming for with the PEW 12 exercise. Here's how it works. Every emotion has a charge, and the positive or negative energy an emotion generates has a real and measurable impact on our bodies. The act of writing allows us to physically release some of that charge much in the same way we release tension during sex. Burning the page, which happens at the end of the exercise, allows us to purge even more of that charge and serves as a symbol of letting go. If you can release negative energy on a regular basis, it doesn't accumulate. You could look at this exercise as an act of freedom. Whenever you release your emotions, you lighten your burden so you don't have to carry it with you to your next experience.

EXERCISE:
Purge Emotional Writing (PEW 12)

This exercise works best if you just keep writing and don't stop to think about what you'll write next or self-edit. Forget about punctuation or making your handwriting pretty, even legible. In fact you may get to the point where your emotions are flowing so fast and furiously that you can't even write real words. That's great. Just keep the pen in contact with the paper and let the thoughts roll out of you. This isn't a time to be polite or fair. This is your side of the story. Also, at the end of the exercise you'll be destroying the pages you've written, so as you write there's no reason to worry about anyone else reading them.

DIRECTIONS

1. Before you begin, get a notebook and pen and find a quiet place where you won't be disturbed. Sit down and set a timer for twelve minutes.
2. Open your notebook and simply start writing about whatever is disturbing your peace. It could be your health, job, finances, personal relationships, or anything else. Don't think about it too much—just start.
3. At the end of twelve minutes, stop writing. Immediately take the pages to a secure, nonflammable area like a concrete patio, your driveway, fireplace, or barbecue and set them on fire. Don't just tear them up. Fire is transformative and cleansing. Your goal is to neutralize the negative energy, and fire does that by changing the chemical composition of the paper to ash.

Things to Remember

- As you finish each writing session, don't read over what you've written! To do this is to reinfect yourself with the negative energy.

- Don't do this on a computer or other electronic device. You want a physical energetic connection between you and the materials you're using—the pen and the paper—so that you can expel as much of the emotional charge as possible. That's why this exercise must be done in your own handwriting.
- You may use lots of powerful, negatively charged words during this process to discharge pain, but remember to *never direct them toward yourself.* Be kind to yourself and know that you have every right to feel what you feel.

Prescription

Do this every day for five days before moving on to the next step. Even after five days, it's a great thing to work into your morning ritual as a way of regularly purging negative energy and maintaining clarity. Think of it as practicing good psycho-spiritual hygiene in the same way you practice good physical hygiene by bathing, grooming, and brushing your teeth.

....

WHY TWELVE?
....

In this exercise, you write for a total of twelve minutes. Why twelve? The number twelve has sacred significance. Many of the world's historical prophets had twelve followers or disciples. Christ fed thousands with five loaves of bread and two fish and had twelve baskets of abundant leftovers. The number also symbolizes balance (there are twelve hours of day and twelve hours of night in a 24-hour period) and the completion of a cycle (we have twelve months before a new year begins).

....

What to Expect from PEW 12

Not long ago my day started with a surprise. Intending to get to my office before anyone else, I was up and out the door early. But when I walked outside, I found something I wasn't expecting. My car, which I'd parked on the street the evening before, was sitting there with the trunk and driver's side door thrown wide open. I stopped dead in my tracks.

I remembered being in a hurry when I arrived home the previous evening, wanting to work on a birthday present I was making for my wife before she got home from her office. Could I have been in such a rush that I'd forgotten to close and lock the car? After a brief moment of confusion, I was certain I hadn't left it that way. Then the obvious answer hit me. My car had been broken into.

I went to survey the damage and, sure enough, some personal items and documents I'd left in the car were missing. As I waited for the police to come so I could file a report, I discovered that my next-door neighbors had a security camera that happened to be pointed in the general direction of my car. I knocked on the door and asked if I could see the recording. While it didn't show my car, it did show the space just behind it. That was where I saw a woman on a bicycle riding away with my belongings. She even dropped a few things as she pedaled away, leaving them on the ground like forgotten and unimportant breadcrumbs.

I couldn't stop thinking about this woman. Her image stuck in my mind. I was angry that she had invaded my space and privacy in such a callous and careless way. I was worried about the personal information she had taken. I was annoyed that my day had been hijacked by an event that was beyond my control. All of these thoughts and feelings were swirling around in my head. In short, I started to stew.

After nearly a day of dwelling on what had happened, I turned to PEW 12. I wanted to stop fixating on my feelings of anger and violation, as well as on the woman who had done this to me. Aware that getting stuck can be a danger to clarity, I began to write. Moving my thoughts and feelings from my inner world to the outer one by putting them on the page helped me get past them and move on from the event. After all my years of practicing PEW 12, I find it still helps me through difficult situations of all kinds, big or small.

So that you aren't left wondering whether PEW 12 is working or if you've somehow done it wrong, it's important to understand the range of reactions you might experience after engaging in the exercise. As long as you follow the directions (i.e., remember to write by hand, don't reread what you've written, etc.), it isn't possible to make a mistake. There's no wrong topic to write about, no wrong words to use, no wrong feelings that might come up as a result of what you're writing.

Afterward you may immediately feel lightened and clearer, or you may feel exhausted and emotionally wrenched. It can be a bit like vomiting from food poisoning. At first you feel achy, tired, and awful, but once you've let it all out you start to feel better. If you keep up the exercise over time, you will eventually feel an emotional shift as your burden of negative energy becomes lighter and lighter with each written page. As with other disciplines such as exercise or meditation, the more you do it, the more benefits you'll see.

Another thing to keep in mind. This is a starting point for processing your emotional waste, so it may bring up emotions that aren't completely purged through the act of writing alone, especially if they've been buried a long time. Don't worry, we're only on step three. Remember to go slowly and aim at making incremental progress. At the moment you're working to clear as much space as possible so you have room to maneuver through the rest of this process.

If thoughts and feelings hang around after completing your cleansing rituals, don't try to suppress or ignore them. Instead try to just sit with them as much as possible. In the steps to come we'll look at how to work with them to learn the lessons they have to teach us before we can fully let them go.

Recognize the Mechanisms of Repression

Now that we have begun to clear our physical and emotional body of negative energy, it's time to look at how we can keep the negativity from building up again. We'll start by bringing awareness to the different methods often used to avoid processing uncomfortable or painful thoughts and feelings.

When we are able to identify what we're feeling in any given moment, then process our emotions as we experience them, we can say we have emotional clarity. Most of us can't achieve emotional clarity because we fear suffering. Suffering leaves us feeling things we don't like to feel. No one likes to feel helpless, victimized, disempowered, guilty, ashamed, enraged, or out of control. Since these are negative feelings, we tend to avoid them at all costs.

Instead of identifying and processing our feelings, we repress them, often burying them deep within. Without realizing it, we may commit these acts of repression not just once, but over and over again. When this pattern continues unchecked, it leads to emotional saturation, an overfilled cup, and an overwhelmed existence.

Patterns of emotional suppression are instinctual and become habitual for many people. If a pattern is ingrained, we can disrupt it in order to bring about greater emotional clarity by becoming more aware of the ways in which we repress our emotions and thus kick-start the pattern. As the 13th-century Persian poet Rumi once wrote, "Your task is not to seek for love, but merely to seek and find all the barriers within yourself that you have built against it."

Most people approach life in the exact opposite way. They decide what they want and go after it. If they want love, they go after it like it's a thing to be won. Going after what you want in life isn't a bad thing, but it's only part of the process of getting what we want. Hot pursuit is the part that focuses on the external, the judgmental realm. But as we've seen, we need to place an equal amount of focus on the internal, imaginal realm. We may expend a lot of effort seeking love, but if there are internal barriers keeping us from receiving it we will always come up empty.

This step is about focusing so that we are able to identify the barriers we erect against becoming clear. When we repress our emotions, they have nowhere to go but inside. This is how we internalize our misunderstandings, misinterpretations, misidentifications, and misperceptions. They then unconsciously direct our behavior and get in our way. They can even alter our sense of reality, convincing us that a trauma we experienced happened in a different way or didn't happen at all. Since to maintain them requires a great deal of effort, they also siphon off a lot of energy. This energy drain leads to anything but clarity. But if we can spot an act of repression, we can do something about it. We can even learn to disrupt old patterns that don't serve us before they can start again.

An act of repression can also be called a protection mechanism. We all use protection mechanisms because they provide a diversion from negative emotions and make us feel strong as we soldier on from one day to the next. Different people use different methods depending on the emotion they want to repress and the way in which they learned to interact with their emotions at an early age. There are three common protection mechanisms people use to repress their emotions. As I explain and give examples of each, consider whether they feel familiar to you. You can also ask yourself the questions at the end of each section to help determine which mechanisms you might be using to avoid processing your own emotional waste.

Emotional Shutdown

It's because unresolved emotional trauma affects our health over time that many of my patients arrive with personal histories as complex and painful as their medical conditions.

This was true of David, a man in his late sixties who was the CEO of one of the largest pharmaceutical companies in the world. He was in critical shape when I first met him, suffering from stage-four prostate cancer that had metastasized to the bone and had been unresponsive to all treatment, including radiation and chemotherapy. Still, he was reluctant to seek new treatment options and came to me only at the behest of one of my previous patients. In fact, one of the first things he said to me was, "I'm only here as a favor to my friend."

From the start David was openly resistant to my questions and any thoughts I tried to share with him. When I began discussing the link between emotional trauma and physical illness, he cut me off, stating flatly, "I haven't had any traumas in my life."

That seemed highly unlikely to me. Everyone experiences trauma at some point, so I explained that trauma is relative to each person. An experience doesn't have to be an act of physical violence for us to be traumatized by it.

As David finally began to share his story over the coming weeks, I could see quite clearly that he had experienced more than his share of trauma. I believed the unresolved emotional issues that resulted were contributing to his cancer and that it was an important part of my role as his physician to help him see this.

For as long as David could remember, he had felt estranged from his mother. She made it clear in a multitude of ways that she preferred his younger brother, who received nearly all her time and affection, whereas she barely acknowledged her oldest son. And on the occasions she did acknowledge him, it usually left a sting.

One day, in front of David and a group of his friends, his mother said, "I know his brother is going to be a great artist someday, but David? I have no idea where he'll end up." His mother's dismissive words cut deeply and only served to confirm the sense of abandonment he had experienced his entire young life. This of course was in addition to the humiliation of having his mother say something so hurtful in front of his friends. Soon after, he was placed in the charge of a nanny who whisked him off to her hometown a continent away, and that was where he did the rest of his growing up.

As an adult, life got better for David, especially after he married Karen, a nurse and supportive wife. They had a beautiful daughter, Grace, and David enjoyed a highly successful career. In spite of his wonderful success, his mother still refused to acknowledge his accomplishments or have any contact with his daughter. "You live so far away," she'd say. "She'll never know me anyway, so why bother?"

One day after returning from a business trip, David was surprised to find his father-in-law and a family friend waiting to pick him up at the airport instead of his usual driver. On the ride home, they gave him the news that while he was away, Karen had died suddenly from an undiagnosed heart condition.

In David's own words, he immediately shut down. Unable to grieve fittingly, he soon packed up all of Karen's belongings and locked them in the attic. Every photograph that bore her image, every video on which he could see her or hear her voice, every greeting card graced with her handwriting was piled into a suitcase and left to linger in the darkness with the rest of his memories of her. At the time, he didn't realize that his actions were yet again being driven by the subconscious pain of feeling unexpectedly abandoned by the most important woman in his life.

There are a number of different ways that people avoid or suppress negative feelings they don't want to feel or don't think they can handle. One of the most common is to simply shut them off. To find an empty room inside ourselves, pack our feelings in there, and lock the door.

The problem is that it's difficult for any of us to shut off some feelings while enjoying a healthy relationship with others. We tend to act more like a faucet in this way. Our emotional faucet is either on or it's off. The feelings either flow through us or they stop moving and become stuck.

When we shut off our feelings, even if we meant to shut off just the unwanted ones, we tend to become emotionally unavailable overall. This leads to relationship problems, loss of interdependency and intimacy, isolation, and sometimes even promiscuity.

David never wanted to look back, so he just kept going. Eventually he sold most of Karen's things, moved to a new city, and remarried. By the time he came to me, which was years after Karen's death, he had been battling cancer for quite some time. He also had a difficult relationship with his daughter, Grace, now in her 30s, whom he described as lazy and overweight. He was concerned that she wasn't dating or making any effort to move forward in her life.

David thought he had escaped the pain of his past when what he'd really done was pack it away and shut the door on it, just like he'd done with the memories of Karen he'd locked away in his attic so many years ago. I told David that in order to heal, he must properly grieve, first for the loss of Karen, then for his mother's love, which had never come. After so many years, he needed to take a trip back to the attic and allow himself the dignity of his own emotional process.

Amazingly, although David had liquidated all of Karen's belongings years before, he still had the suitcase with all of her photos, videos, and cards. In an incredible act of bravery, he began to view the old home movies and pictures of Karen and open the cards she'd given him to read her beautiful words. It was only a week or so after he'd done this that he called to tell me how, for the first time ever, his cancer was responding to treatment.

These positive results inspired David to unearth even more buried emotions. His mother had passed away by then, but he used the PEW 12 exercise to talk to her in his own way, writing out a dialogue between them as if he was writing a script. He then burned the pages, helping him release long-held negative feelings toward her. As a bonus, even his relationship with Grace and his current wife benefited from his emotional and energetic shift.

All the while, his prostate continued to shrink. It didn't happen overnight, but his oncologist has officially declared him to be in remission as he continues to do the work of honoring his emotional process in all areas of his life. I don't believe any of this would have happened had David not allowed himself to turn his emotional faucet back on and fully process the loss of love from two of the most important women in his life.

ARE YOU EMOTIONALLY SHUT DOWN?

If you answer yes to most or all of the following questions, it may be a sign you have emotionally shut down.

1. Do you have trouble admitting you experience negative feelings or that you have suffered trauma in your life?

2. Do you avoid emotionally charged situations or conversations?
3. Do you keep all or most of the people in your life at arm's length, never or rarely achieving true closeness and intimacy?
4. Do you often feel isolated or alone?
5. Do you engage in promiscuous behavior?

Emotional Posturing

Shutting down so we don't have to feel at all is one way in which we avoid uncomfortable emotions. Another is to pretend that the emotions aren't there, that they aren't all that important, or that they've already been dealt with when they haven't. This is emotional posturing, which often shows up in our lives as a story we tell ourselves and others that explains why we are ignoring or minimizing our own feelings. "It really wasn't all that bad," we assure ourselves. Or we tell ourselves, "It's okay because it's all in the past. I'm really over it by now."

In the case of my patient Mark, his method of minimizing his feeling was to say, "It was such a long time ago, it really doesn't matter anymore."

Despite being only in his mid-40s, Mark hadn't worked for seven years because he suffered from intractable pain in his right leg. The pain was so severe that he was on twelve separate prescription medications, including the narcotic painkiller Percocet, an anti-anxiety medication, and even an anti-psychotic. When he described the pain, he said it was constant whenever he was lying down or seated. Curiously, it subsided only when he was walking or moving forward.

It was as if a dark cloud enveloped Mark whenever he talked about his pain. Except that the cloud seemed to go away when he talked about his family. He had been married to Nicole, an executive at an international entertainment conglomerate, for 18 years. They had two children, an 11-year-old son and a 14-year-old daughter. He clearly adored them.

I saw something change in his behavior, however, when I asked him if anything significant had happened in his life seven years ago, around the time his leg pain had started. He didn't take long to respond: "Nicole and I were having problems then because I suspected she was having an affair with someone at work."

When I tried to obtain more information concerning this revelation, Mark quickly tried to pass it off as "no big deal." I persisted until finally he confessed, "You know, it's not like I haven't done a lot of rotten things in my life too. I cheated on my first wife, so I have to forgive Nicole even though she never admitted to anything. It was such a long time ago, it really doesn't matter anymore. I let it go so we could move forward."

"But Mark, I don't believe you've let it go," I told him as gently as I could. "That's why you're still in pain. This pain began shortly after you suspected your wife of cheating on you. Instead of confronting her and working through your feelings, you used the guilt from your first marriage to talk yourself out of going through a proper emotional process. You may have cheated on your first wife, but that has no bearing on your relationship with Nicole. You've convinced yourself you don't have a right to your feelings, so your pain and anger have gone unexpressed. The only way to truly stand up and move forward with your life isn't to bypass your feelings and pretend they're not there, but to acknowledge and process them openly and fully."

Mark was silent. I could tell he was thinking about what I'd said, but he hadn't responded beyond a few *uh-huh*s and *okay*s. I decided to take a different tack.

"Mark," I said, "I know your family is very important to you. I can understand why you would never want to risk losing them, even if it meant denying your feelings and suffering physical pain because of it. Unfortunately that's not helping you move forward. It's keeping your marriage stuck and you in pain. Eventually those unexpressed issues between you and Nicole will grow and jeopardize the survival of your family anyway."

Mark remained quiet and after a little while ended our conversation by promising to think about what I'd said. A few days later I received an email from him thanking me for my services and stating that he was ending our professional relationship because he believed we weren't "the right fit."

At the time, Mark wasn't ready to take the steps he needed to take in order to bring clarity to his situation, and that's okay. Growth is a process and sometimes we have false starts or detours along the way. Mark did return to my office a year later after having tried more extreme treatments, from pain blockers to morphine, all of which failed to alleviate his suffering. We are now working through these steps together and he's gradually learning to face his feelings. I believe he and his relationship will begin to heal once he stops pretending his feelings don't matter.

....

ARE YOU EMOTIONALLY POSTURING?

....

If you answer yes to most or all of the following questions, it may be a sign you are emotionally posturing.

1. Do you often diminish the importance of your feelings when talking about them (e.g., "It doesn't really matter anymore")?
2. Do you often diminish the magnitude of your feelings when talking about them (e.g., "It wasn't all that bad")?
3. Do you often try to put on a happy face about things or look on the bright side?
4. Do you find that your negative feelings come out in ways you weren't expecting?

5. Have you been taking one or more prescription medications over an extended period for conditions like pain, insomnia, anxiety, or depression?

....

Emotional Armoring

Emotional armoring is the act of putting up barriers between ourselves and others. This happens when we see ourselves as victims and someone or something outside of us as the cause or potential cause of our pain. As a result we armor ourselves against the outside threat in order to make ourselves feel safe and protected.

I witnessed a pronounced case of emotional armoring when Laura came to my office looking for help shedding the significant amount of weight she had gained over the previous two years. It had gotten to the point where the weight was impeding her job performance as a corrections officer in the men's wing of the county jail.

Only 32 years old, Laura initially believed that with enough effort she would be able to get back down to a more manageable weight on her own. But after diets, exercise regimens, and other interventions failed to work, she began to suspect a hormonal problem. I ordered a hormone panel to check her theory. When it came back normal, I started looking into other aspects of her life.

As I got to know Laura better, I discovered she hadn't been in a relationship for several years. At first she didn't want to talk about it, insisting she just hadn't felt like pursuing a relationship. But something told me this was an important area to discuss. I continued asking questions about her past romantic relationships such as, *When was your last long-term relationship? What was it like? Why did it end? Have you tried to start a new relationship since then? Have you been on any dates?* Little by little Laura began to open up, until finally she revealed she had been sexually assaulted prior to taking her job as a corrections officer. The assault had ended any desire for a romantic relationship, which is why she hadn't tried to pursue one since.

After hearing this, I politely suggested to Laura that her inexplicable weight gain might be a subconscious protection mechanism to keep men, whom she now felt were dangerous, away by making herself unattractive to them. At the same time, the job she'd taken as a corrections officer in a men's jail following her assault suggested a subconscious need to be in a position of authority over men in a place where she could see bad guys being punished. With access to a gun and the men securely behind bars, she gained an additional sense of safety. Not only had she shielded herself from others, she had shielded herself from her own uncomfortable emotions such as fear and shame. Only after she learned to identify this pattern could she begin to make changes in her life and lose the weight.

Once Laura understood this, I put her on a detox protocol and worked with her to express her repressed emotions. As part of her treatment, she went on the Intentional Unsaturation Diet and learned the same PEW 12 exercise we covered in the previous step. She returned to her normal weight over the course of the next eighteen months.

ARE YOU EMOTIONALLY ARMORING?

If you answer yes to most or all of the following questions, it may be a sign you are emotionally armoring.

1. Do you often avoid situations that make you feel uncomfortable, vulnerable, or exposed?
2. Do you find yourself making excuses for why you can't pursue what you want in life even though you can't possibly know the outcome for sure (e.g., "I can't be in a relationship,

because with all the extra weight I'm carrying no one will ever find me attractive" or, "I'm terrible at interviews, so I can never quit my job. I'll never get a new one.")?

3. Do you often avoid telling people what you really think?

4. Do you tend to conceal your true self from others for fear they won't like or accept you?

5. Do you often feel disconnected from your emotional self, or like there is a barrier between you and it?

....

Becoming Aware

No matter what mechanism we use to try to separate ourselves from our feelings, repressed emotions may be out of sight but never out of mind. If we ignore them, they simply find new, more emphatic ways to express themselves, be it through weight gain, depression, anxiety, unhappiness, dissatisfaction, stress, pain, or any number of illnesses. Whatever the issue, we certainly can't heal if we avoid it altogether or take an adversarial position and fight it.

For now your task is to simply notice which of the mechanisms you may be using in your life or may have used in the past, so that you begin creating an awareness of your patterns and habits. Bringing awareness to your relationship with your emotions may sound like a small step, but it's actually huge. Once you can spot a pattern, you can work to change it. Knowing that you are judgmental in certain situations gives you the opportunity to change your approach. Knowing that certain people or situations cause you fear helps you find ways to transcend those fears. As odd as it may sound, you can think of this like a treasure hunt. Spotting the ways in which you avoid uncomfortable or painful emotions is the first clue on your hunt.

Next you're going to learn how to ask questions that will enable you to follow the signs your mind and body send you, so that you can go back to their source in the emotions you are keeping buried. The point of this is to bring these emotions into the light where they can be accorded the dignity of proper acknowledgment that they deserve. Once they're uncovered, you can learn the lessons they have to teach you. Remember the story of the golden Buddha. Every mishap, every crack in your surface is just another opportunity to find the golden treasure hidden underneath.

Follow the Signs

Now that you have learned how you might be avoiding difficult emotions, you want to begin looking past the mechanisms of repression to the emotions themselves—what they are, where they came from, and why you felt the need to repress them in the first place.

In this step I'm going to describe how to use the clues you are given to look inward, which can be harder than it sounds. The reason this can be tricky is because every one of us has perceptual constraints that cause us to see what we *want* to see or what makes sense to us based on our past experiences, rather than what's actually there. To get a better sense of what I mean, read the following example:

Paris
in the
the spring

When you read this, did you notice the extra *the*? Or did you read *Paris in the spring*? Most people see the latter for the simple reason that the sentence makes more sense without the second *the*. Often people have trouble seeing the extra word even when they've been prompted to look closely. (If you're having difficulty seeing it, look at both the second and the third lines.) We've been taught to trust what we see with our own eyes, but this small example shows how easily our vision is influenced by our perception. As I pointed out earlier, reality is irrelevant and perception is everything because it's our perception that guides us in real life situations.

Let's look at another example. Read the following sentence and think about what it means to you:

Woman without her man is incomplete.

Did this sentence make you angry? If so, why? Now look at the variations of the sentence that follow and see if you change your mind:

Woman, without her man, is incomplete.
Woman, without her, man is incomplete.

The first sentence suggests that a woman needs a man. The second suggests exactly the opposite, that man needs a woman. The meaning of the sentence changes completely as a result of the placement of the comma. The first version of the sentence has no commas at all, yet most people I show it to read one of these two meanings into it all the same. Because the sentence isn't clear as written, people tend to project their own meaning onto it, a meaning based on their own experiences. Which meaning they choose reveals something about how they perceive the dynamic between men and women. In much the same way, unless we have clarity our perceptions tend to be colored by our past experiences and the preconceived judgments, limiting beliefs, and misidentifications that often result.

If it's so easy to misperceive short sentences like these or to have them colored by our past experiences, imagine how easy it would be with something more complex like our emotional selves or the world around us. It's important to keep this in mind as you continue on this journey.

The hardships we've endured in our lives leave us with guilt, shame, anger, and resentment. These negative feelings cloud our vision and keep us unconsciously thinking and acting in ways that may be counter to who we are and what we want. So much of this happens beneath the surface unconsciously. Without even realizing it, we developed patterns long ago that we still follow even if doing so isn't in our best interest.

So how do you spot your misperceptions if they happen unconsciously? This is a crucial question because even slight misperceptions get in the way of clarity. Real self-knowledge, by which I mean being able to see ourselves and the situations in our lives clearly and without preconceived judgments, is essential for clarity.

The way you will find them is by paying attention and following the signs. Your consciousness will always send you clues that you can follow back to the source. These clues, or signals, are the projections that were discussed in chapter 2. Remember, the way we perceive everything in our outer world is a projection of some part of our inner reality. This means that any mental or physical issue that manifests itself in our external life can be mined for the corresponding issue inside us.

Monitoring Our Energy Levels

Every time we make an inauthentic choice, that choice ripples through the body. An example might be agreeing to go out with friends when we're not really interested in where they're going. The negative feelings and misperceptions that result from an inauthentic choice (in this case, the feeling of "I really don't want to be doing this") activate the autonomic nervous system, the part of our nervous system that regulates involuntary functions like digestion and heart rate. In other words, our negative feelings actually trigger a measurable physiological response, which can consist of a rise in blood pressure, an accelerated heart rate, faster breathing, and constricted blood vessels. This taxes the body, literally draining it of energy and making it harder for us to resist outside pressure.

David R. Hawkins, MD, PhD, came up with an exercise based on this idea that can be a great way to test whether you are thinking clearly and responding authentically to an issue or situation. It's called the muscle test and it's quite easy to do:

1. Stand opposite a friend and hold your right arm out to the side. Speak out loud a statement about what you believe is affecting you in the current moment. You might say, "I love my job."

2. After you've spoken, your friend, with moderate effort, will try to push your arm back down to your side with one hand as you try to resist. If the statement is true for you, your arm will remain strong and in place. If the statement is false on any level, your arm will go weak and be pushed down to your side no matter how hard you try to resist.

You may be skeptical about this exercise, but think about how it feels when you really don't want to do something. Maybe you have a chore you've been putting off or someone you don't particularly like whom you need to call. What does it feel like when you think about those things? Do you feel tired, listless, deflated?

The reason we feel such things is that it takes effort to bury our feelings and to employ the protection mechanisms that keep them buried. The more effort we expend on suppressing our feelings, the less energy we have for other things like resisting outside pressures or engaging in activities we truly enjoy. If we tune into how our energy ebbs and flows, we can pinpoint what's happening or what we're doing in moments when it feels like our energy is being sapped.

As you spend more time with this process and gain clarity, it will become easier to perceive subtle shifts in energy. In the beginning, however, it will likely be the larger shifts that get your attention. When we make lots of inauthentic choices over time, they add up and take a toll. Disease is a metaphor for what's happening at the soul level, and what saps our energy more than a major illness of the mind or body? Whether it's stress, depression, or cancer, what these things have in common is that they rob us of positive energy. When you perceive any shift in energy, no matter how big or small, consider it a clue to look inside for the emotions associated with this shift.

Monitoring Where You Feel Your Emotions

I've mentioned how patients often describe their upset in physical terms: "He's such a pain in the neck" or, "I can't stomach this situation any longer." This is no accident. Researchers in Finland actually mapped various emotions in the body through a series of experiments ("Bodily Maps of Emotions," PNAS, November 27, 2013). Different regions of the body registered either an increase or decrease in energy based on the emotion a person was feeling. The findings suggest that different emotions may well be associated with different sensations in the body.

Anger, for example, showed up in the head and arms, which makes sense when you think about it. A tightening of the fists and a flushed face are symptoms often associated with anger. In contrast, disgust was felt in the throat and digestive tract, as if feeling disgusted by a person or idea could literally cause someone to feel sick to their stomach. Depression, on the other hand, registered as either a lack of or decrease in feeling throughout much of the body, especially in a person's head and extremities.

For those of us who may have trouble identifying our feelings, monitoring our bodily sensations when we are emotionally triggered may help us understand and articulate what we're experiencing. This can also be useful for helping us see past our mechanisms of repression. For instance, someone who is emotionally shut down may not admit to feeling anxious even though they are experiencing a tightness or pressure in their chest. Consult the following chart to see whether you recognize where in the body your emotions might be living.

··

EMOTIONS AND THE BODY

··

Anger: Hotheaded, tightened fists, and an increased heart rate. Anger tends to register as heat spreading from the chest throughout the upper body, including the head and arms.

Depression: A lack of energy, especially in the limbs and head. Depression can show up as grogginess and a disinclination to move, to get up and go.

Sadness: Like depression, sadness often manifests as a lack of energy in the arms and legs. Unlike depression, there's a simultaneous increase in energy around the eyes, in the throat, and in the chest, the same areas that are affected by crying.

Disgust: Feeling like something is caught in your throat or like you want to vomit. When someone feels disgusted, it's as if they literally can't digest the feeling they are experiencing.

Anxiety: Often felt as a tightness or pressure in the chest. Anxiety appears like a tight ball of excess energy sitting around the heart.

Shame: Flushed cheeks and chest, a queasiness in the stomach. The extra energy in these regions is matched by a decrease of energy in the limbs, as if the person is stuck, unable to move.

Happiness: A warm glow throughout the body, with extra activation in the head and upper chest.

Love: A warm glow throughout the body, with extra activation through the chest and groin.

Asking Questions

Drops in energy tend to be accompanied by negative feelings. Maybe you're feeling tired and sluggish in the mornings. Could it be because you feel a sense of dread about going to work? Maybe you get angry when your spouse asks you for a simple favor either because you're already overwhelmed with your schedule or because the last time you asked for a favor yourself, he or she said no, which made you feel upset and uncared for.

Clarity requires you to do something that may not feel natural to you at first. Anytime you encounter a negative feeling ("I *dread* going to work," "I *hate* my job" or, "My partner is *ticking me off*"), you are likely to want to repress it through one of the mechanisms we talked about in the last chapter. We do this because none of us enjoys feeling bad. Yet ignoring our feelings isn't going to get us anywhere. Not only is it not going to help us deepen our understanding of ourselves, it's not even going to make us feel better in the long run. Remember, feelings buried alive never die. The best thing we can do is to simply stop and sit with the feeling for a moment. Then, instead of turning away, tune in.

When these energetic shifts happen and the negative feelings occur, these are clues to start asking open-ended questions. *What*

*is it about my job that I don't love? Why have I stayed in this job if I
don't love it? Why haven't I admitted to myself before this moment that
I don't love my job? What would I rather be doing instead?*

If what you're feeling is part of a pattern (i.e., it isn't just this job
you don't like, but the last one and the one before that as well), you
can ask yourself even more questions. *What about me keeps attract-
ing this kind of situation into my life? How did I contribute to creating
this unhappy pattern?*

Of course, if we're not careful, asking questions can lead back to
the same preconceived judgments and limiting beliefs we're trying
to interrupt and see past. For example, if you ask someone why she
doesn't like her job, she could easily answer, "It's my boss' fault. He's
such a jerk! I can't stand the way he talks to me."

If this is the kind of answer you receive, you need to continue
asking questions until you get back to *you* and *your relationship*
to the situation. This is because everything in our life is really all
about us—our beliefs, our feelings, our perceptions, our choices.
These are the things that got us where we are today. Yes, things
happen that are beyond our control and people do things to us we
wouldn't have chosen. We can't control what others do, and neither
can we prevent other people's actions from affecting us, but this
doesn't render us powerless. We can still self-parent and choose to
process the emotions that arise as a result of what happens in the
way that best serves us.

We can also choose how we want to frame those events in our
minds. In this book you are working toward a place where you
choose to frame yourselves and your circumstances in ways that
best support the kind of life you want and the kind of person you
truly are. This requires you to understand the part *you* play in every
situation, as well as the fact you always have the power to choose
how to respond.

For example, if you don't like your boss, then the questions might be, *Why have I stayed so long in this job if my boss is so terrible? If other people aren't bothered by my boss like I am, what is he triggering in me that he's not triggering in them? What signals do I give off that make my boss think it's okay to be disrespectful when he speaks to me? When my boss speaks disrespectfully to me, why haven't I spoken up about it or done anything to change it? Don't I believe I have the power to change how people treat me?*

There are two important things to keep in mind as you ask yourself questions about what you're feeling:

1. Keep the focus on how *you* are contributing to your circumstances.
2. Just because you are focusing on yourself doesn't mean you are blaming yourself. You're simply looking for information and insight, so keep an open mind without preconceived judgments or blame.

For this kind of self-evaluation to be effective, there needs to be no blaming, no self-judgment. This means not blaming others such as your boss, and equally important not blaming yourself. Neither option will help you move forward.

What will help you move forward is coming to the realization that you have such a strong reaction to your boss because he reminds you of your father, for whom nothing you did ever seemed good enough. Or you many discover that you take unwanted job after unwanted job because you are afraid to pursue the kind of position you really want because you're afraid you're not good enough to get it. These kinds of realizations aren't to be avoided or feared, but on the contrary are a reason to celebrate since they reveal beliefs you can then work to change for the better (which I will help you do in the steps that follow).

EXERCISE:
Asking Open-Ended Questions

When asking yourself the kind of questions that will help you uncover the inner issue that corresponds to the outer clues you're following, it can help to imagine a conversation between two parts of yourself—the part that exists in the outer judgmental realm and the part that exists in the inner imaginal realm, which I've previously referred to as the authentic self.

As you facilitate a dialogue between these two parts, it's important to ask the right questions so you can get to the root of the issue, open windows to new realizations and ideas, and prevent the conversation from being shut down by the judgmental self.

Things to Remember

Asking open-ended questions

- creates a safe environment where unconscious thoughts and feelings are given permission to surface
- allows you to express yourself more freely and completely
- invites relevant and meaningful exploration of the issues
- offers the judgmental self the opportunity to discover its own solution in an organic way, while experiencing the validation of speaking its truth.

DIRECTIONS

1. Begin by calling in your authentic self in the same way that you did for the intention-setting exercise on page 60.

2. For the moment, let go of any notions of what you believe you "should" do or feel about the present situation.

3. Avoid closed-ended questions—questions that tend to lead to a yes-or-no answer and don't offer opportunities to explain. For example:

   • Do you get along well with your spouse?
   • Is your job satisfying to you?
   • Does money play a part in your marriage problems?

4. Avoid leading questions that tell your judgmental self what to think. For example:

   • Why is my husband such a jerk?
   • Do I really think my ex-husband forgot about visitation or did he just want to hurt us?
   • Do I really believe what she said about my invitation to the party getting lost in the mail?

5. Ask questions of the judgmental self respectfully and listen receptively from your authentic self. For example:

   • Why do I think my partner has pulled away from me sexually?
   • How did our relationship change after we got married?
   • What is it about my work that I find so challenging?
   • What's my earliest memory of my mother acting in this way that I find hurtful?
   • What did I learn from the experience and how can it help me now?

Helpful Hint: At first it can help to differentiate between your two selves—the authentic self and judgmental self—in the dialogue by setting up two chairs facing each other. When commenting as the judgmental self, sit in one chair. When ready to reply as the authentic self, switch to the other chair. For some this helps to switch between mindsets and thus facilitates the conversation.

No Matter How Bad It May Seem...

I'm usually the doctor patients come to after they've exhausted other options. This means I see my fair share of patients who are suffering from very serious, advanced, or rare medical conditions. Because I believe biography dictates biology, they often arrive in my office with highly complex and painful personal histories to match.

By the time 42-year-old Macy came to me, she was suffering an extremely rare condition in which her vaginal tissue had become sclerotic, meaning it had thinned out and turned extremely dry and rigid. This stiffening of such normally supple tissue causes severe chronic pain and makes intercourse impossible. The appointment with Macy started with taking her medical history and learning about the long list of treatment options she'd tried. Then I asked her when her symptoms first showed up.

"My present condition started a few months ago," she explained, "but prior to that I'd been having recurring urinary infections for quite some time."

"Do you know what prompted those infections?"

"I can't say for sure, but they occurred following each time I had sex with my husband."

That was my clue to begin discussing her primary relationship. After several questions about the nature of their relationship, she finally revealed that it was often "very difficult."

"Difficult in what way?" I prompted her.

"He has a short temper. It doesn't take much for him to fly into a rage and say terrible things to me."

"What sorts of things?"

"He tells me I'm not worth all the money he spends on me. He's a Wall Street broker who makes a very good living, so it's not like he can't afford it."

"Anything else?"

"Sometimes he tells me I'm stupid or that he doesn't know why he married me."

"He's verbally abusive to you."

"I guess."

"Has anyone else been abusive to you in the past?" Macy looked at me for a moment and then nodded.

"More than one person?" She looked at me again and nodded.

"Can you tell me about the first person you remember abusing you?"

I've heard many heartbreaking histories over the course of my career, but this question kicked off a story that was more than even I was prepared for. Macy grew up in an affluent household with a stay-at-home mother and a father who enjoyed a successful career. Although everything in the household looked practically perfect from the outside, Macy was quietly struggling. She secretly yearned for the attention and affection of her father, who simply refused to acknowledge her in any meaningful way. On the rare occasion he took notice of her, it was usually to verbally and physically abuse her in much the same way he abused her mother.

As Macy grew up, she felt increasingly like she was an inconvenience to her socially active parents. In order to fill her time while they were off doing other things, her parents suggested she start dating a 19-year-old man whose parents they'd recently become acquainted with. She was just twelve at the time.

Macy's parents didn't seem to mind that Mike would pick her up on his motorcycle, fly down the highways at nearly 100 miles per hour with her on the back, or return her late in the evenings. For Macy, it was all a rush and she enjoyed feeling like Mike cared about her.

Until one evening, when Mike returned her home. Having said hello to her mother, who was in the kitchen with the cook, he insisted on seeing Macy's room. She led him upstairs, and while her mother was downstairs overseeing dinner preparations, he raped her in her own bed. Soon after he left the house as if nothing had happened. Traumatized, Macy sat through dinner with her parents, never mentioning what had happened.

Macy said she lost all respect for herself after that. By high school she had become highly promiscuous. At 16, she convinced her father to send her on his private jet to the university she wanted to attend to experience Greek Week. While there, she offered herself up to one man after another, each of whom treated her with the same disregard she felt for herself.

After high school her destructive pattern continued. She moved from partner to partner and developed issues with alcohol and self-mutilation. She was still in her twenties when she moved to New York City, where she met her husband, Rick. Many nights after they married, she found herself wondering about the similarities between her childhood and adult life.

Since she had always been treated with disregard and abuse, she figured she must deserve it on some level. She'd spent her life reaching out to men for love and they always ended up rejecting her, a pattern that left her with the unconscious belief that love is punishment—punishment she deserved.

After hearing this, I formed the opinion that Macy's vaginal sclerosis was her body's way of armoring her against further abuse from yet another man in her life, since she physically couldn't have sex any longer.

In addition to Macy's medical protocol, I worked extensively with her to help her understand that although her biological father rejected her, there was a Higher Power that could provide guidance and love her the way she needed. She learned how to connect to this Higher Power, as well as how to release much of the pain and anger she'd been holding against her mother for not doing more to protect her—and even more strongly against her father, her husband, the boyfriend who had raped her, and so many other men in her life. She worked on reframing her idea of men and masculinity as something other than damaging and dangerous. And she came to believe that real love from men was possible and something she deserved to experience.

It's rare to see patients put so much effort into their recovery, especially when faced with multiple serious traumas over so many years. But Macy was determined to reclaim her life, and she did. She and I worked together for a year and a half. I helped her understand that she didn't need to continue carrying the burden of her past with her into her future and showed her how to purge the negative energy she had been storing.

We also worked on ways she could be more open and honest about what she had been through, rather than hiding in shame. When she finally told Rick the whole story, he was shocked. Nineteen years together and he had no idea. Although she had always felt damaged by her past, as if people would reject her if they knew, the fact that Rick not only accepted what she told him but loved her all the more for letting him in was a truly healing experience for both of them.

By the end of our time together, Macy's vaginal sclerosis had completely healed. She has no more urinary tract infections either, so she went off all her medications, including her antibiotics. Her marriage to Rick improved, and best of all she felt newly able to guide her young daughters into making self-affirming choices in life and love.

Keep Searching

Searching for clues and asking the kind of questions that will bring buried emotions to the surface isn't always easy. You may find that when you try the exercise of asking open-ended questions, you don't get very far. That's all right. It doesn't mean you've failed or that the process isn't going to work for you. Remember, it's important to go slowly and be kind to yourself along the way.

You should always keep asking questions. If it doesn't work today, try again tomorrow. If you're persistent, one day the answers will find their way to the surface. The more you do this, the easier it will get to access your feelings and process them. If this isn't reason enough to keep at it, know that the source of your pain or discomfort won't go away until it has been dealt with properly, which is why I encourage you to try and try again.

The ultimate goal here is to get to a place in your life where you don't have to wait for a major illness or crisis to get your attention. There's a state of consciousness in which you can process and clear your emotions while they're happening, and that's what you're aiming for. You don't have to wait for more pronounced signals. Each time you take the opportunity to follow a signal to its source and process what you find with care, you clear more space inside you. What's more, the process of creating clarity becomes more familiar, less scary and daunting, and easier to work through the next time you need it.

What to Do with Doubt and Fear

When we don't understand how our emotions create our circumstances, we can feel as if life just happens to us. Feeling disempowered fills us with uncertainty and apprehension about the future. It leaves us unable to trust the process of life. We doubt that we already have within us everything we need to see us through any situation.

When we are filled with doubt, we feel vulnerable. This causes us to act like victims whose only choices are to fight back against what's threatening us or run from it. This is the opposite of the holistic view we need for clarity. Instead of seeing the mind and the body as parts of the same whole, instead of cycling continuously between the inner imaginal and outer judgmental realms, embracing the ebb and the flow of life, we either pit one part of ourselves or our world against the other or we prioritize one part over the other. This leaves us feeling anything but whole. Instead we become split. In fact, the word *doubt* comes from the word *double*, implying a splitting process.

Chances are you've experienced some doubts already as you've worked your way through the initial steps in this process. I've pointed out a few places where doubt might have come up. When you were asked to eat differently on the Intentional Unsaturation Diet, for example, did you doubt whether it was possible for you to give up caffeine, eat sardines for breakfast, or put your vegetarianism on hold for a few days? Did you doubt whether it was even a good idea? When asked to mine your feelings for insights in the last step, did you doubt whether you could truly face your greatest traumas? Did you wonder whether it wouldn't be better to leave them buried where they are? When I first introduced the idea of clarity and what it can do, did you doubt that change on the scale I've suggested was even possible for you? For anyone?

Doubts are natural, but they are also barriers that keep us from moving forward. You may doubt you can handle facing your traumas, but how can you be sure until you try? You may doubt you can eat a certain way, but isn't that really an artificial barrier you've created? You may doubt you can stick to a daily habit of doing your PEW 12 writing exercises, but what is the harm in giving it a shot? When we give in to our doubts, we miss opportunities to expand our world and through doing so discover more about who we truly are.

Think about it this way. If you relax your eyes to the point where you are seeing double, what happens? Things get blurry and you lose focus. When you are seeing clearly, it's because the brain takes the two images you are seeing through each of your two eyes and combines them into one. Just as double vision causes us to lose focus, so also does doubt. It keeps us from becoming clear. That's why in this step we're going to discuss how to deal with the inevitable doubts that arise, as well as the fears that often follow in doubt's wake.

The Relationship between Doubt and Fear

Fear is caused by doubt. When we're comfortable with who we are and what we're experiencing, we don't feel fear. Instead we tend to go on our merry way without thinking too much about it. However, when we feel discomfort because we're dealing with the unknown, our doubt leads us to second-guess not only ourselves but even our circumstances. We begin to imagine, *What if?* We wonder about all the things that might happen, often to the point of scaring ourselves. As I like to say to my patients, "Our lives are filled with terrible misfortunes, most of which never happen."

If doubt morphs into fear, the fear leaves us feeling stuck, unable to move and make changes in our lives. Clarity requires movement, a natural ebb and flow, so being stuck is incompatible with clarity. What we often fail to understand is that doubt and fear originate *within* us.

Certain external events can trigger fear. If there's a fire in your home, it will cause you to feel fear, and that fear will help you get out of there quickly, which is good. However, in our modern society most of the fears we face aren't triggered by something external like a fire. They're triggered by something internal, something imagined, such as the doubts we have about ourselves and our environment. This means we unintentionally create many of our own "terrible misfortunes"—which is precisely why it's so important that we learn how to *contain* our doubts. When they get away from us, the consequences can be tragic.

I once had a patient who reluctantly admitted to me that he'd been living a lie for 30 years. As a young man, he had applied for an executive-level engineering position in a major firm. He really wanted the job but doubted he could get it on his own merit, so he used a friend's résumé and college transcripts. He got the job, thrived in the position, and gradually made his way up the corporate ladder. But time didn't lessen his burden. On the contrary, with each promotion his fear that someone would find him out intensified, as did his guilt and the feeling that he didn't deserve what he had.

In three decades with the firm no one ever discovered his secret. He safely retired from his job, but not from the misery that came with it. His career-long deception had left him, as he described it, "feeling like shit every day."

Of course, this man didn't come to me because he was feeling guilty and afraid his deception would be revealed. He came to see me because he had malignant melanoma that had spread to his lungs, liver, and bones. His condition didn't surprise me when I heard his story. In my experience, people who feel soiled in some way often develop skin cancers. That this man's cancer had spread to his bones signaled the lack of personal integrity involved in his deception.

His self-doubt, manifested in his doubt about being good enough to get the job he wanted, had metastasized just like his cancer. He was petrified that someone would learn the truth about him after all this time. What would they think of him? How could they ever forgive him? His situation was further complicated by the fact that admitting his deception could have resulted in legal action being taken by his firm and the loss of his sizable retirement package. He couldn't fathom doing that to either his family or himself. No wonder he felt stuck, as if there was no way out of his untenable situation.

It's amazing to think that all of this started with one small moment of self-doubt. With every year that passed, it became harder and harder for him to change his circumstances, until the situation was nearly impossible. We talked it through and I finally asked him if he might consider a kind of compromise. I suggested he keep the secret from his past employer but be truthful with his wife. I pointed out that he'd taken a chance once before in deceiving his employer, so he might consider taking a chance once more, this time concerning the idea that he was worth forgiving. After much agonizing he finally agreed to tell her.

Although it was a shock to his wife, she was eventually able to understand and empathize. Forgiveness didn't happen all at once, but they are working through the issues. The patient and I continue to work together as well, but full healing will continue to require the toughest of choices. The good news is that after doing some of this work he's still alive—four years after his oncologist had given him less than a year to live.

There's Doubt, and Then There's Doubt

What can be done about our doubts, especially given that they have the potential to grow into such an overwhelming burden?

The first thing to understand about doubt is that there are two kinds. The first is *unhealthy self-doubt,* which is to have such doubts about yourself and your circumstances that you feel compelled to unconsciously make choices that don't serve you. This kind of doubt is the biggest barrier to clarity.

But doubt in and of itself isn't bad. In fact there is a form of *healthy self-doubt* that's essential for clarity. To understand the difference between unhealthy and healthy doubt, imagine you're a warrior going into battle. If you're absolutely certain your enemy is going to advance in a particular manner and from a particular direction, you leave yourself open to a sneak attack. The warrior who uses his uncertainty to be ready for anything can adapt to changing and unforeseen circumstances, which means he lives to see another day.

Healthy self-doubt comes from accepting a situation as it is without needing to fill in all the blanks or know all the answers right off the bat. It's allowing for uncertainty and accepting you don't know everything. It's being okay with the unknown, which allows you to move forward rather than being stuck in indecisiveness or held back by your fears.

The English Romantic poet John Keats called this the concept of negative capability, which is the ability to sit with the mystery of life and trust the process. He once wrote a letter to his brothers in which he talked about how the idea came to him while he was walking with two acquaintances:

Several things dove-tailed in my mind, and at once it struck me, what quality went to form a Man of Achievement especially in Literature & which Shakespeare possessed so enormously— I mean *Negative Capability*, that is when a man is capable of being in uncertainties, Mysteries, doubts, without any irritable reaching after fact & reason.

In the story I just told about my patient and his career-long lie, a dose of healthy self-doubt would have led him to apply for the job he wanted using his own résumé and transcripts, then trusting the process. Even if he didn't get that particular job, he could have believed in his ability to handle rejection and move on. He could have reassured himself this wasn't the only suitable position in the world and he would find one that was right for him if things didn't turn out the way he wanted. Maybe this would mean acquiring additional education or work experience. Trusting that he could figure out what he needed to do, and that he was capable of doing it, would have made all the difference. Surely it would have been better than a lifetime of deceit.

Doubt will never be completely absent from our lives. Think of it in terms of a spectrum. On the left you hold a lot of unhealthy self-doubt, whereas on the right you enjoy a state of being in which you embody healthy self-doubt. The latter is like being in the eye of a hurricane, where it's completely still. It's in the still place within you, where healthy doubt resides, that you are able to make conscious decisions to improve your circumstances.

Of course, this is a lifelong process and no one can truly stay in this state permanently, so the goal is to continually move in this direction. The more you can let go of unhealthy self-doubt and live comfortably with a sense of healthy self-doubt, the greater the clarity you will have. The exercises that follow will help you move in the right direction.

EXERCISE:
What Then?

On a healing journey, many scare themselves unnecessarily with wild stories of what might happen to them or questions that revolve around *What if?* Fear and doubt impede emotional healing, which is why this exercise is designed to prove that in so many cases our fears are phantoms. When we pull the sheet away there's really nothing there.

DIRECTIONS

1. Sit down with a notepad and pen and write at the top of a blank page what's frightening you or something you have doubts about.
2. On the line below write, "What then?"
3. Think about that question for a moment, then write down the answer.
4. On the line below your answer, once again write, "What then?" Think about it, then write down your answer.
5. Keep this back-and-forth going until you whittle your doubt and fear down to practically nothing.

Example

The exercise might go something like this:

I'm afraid that if I confront my father about the abuse, he'll disinherit me.
What then?
I won't have any money for my future.
What then?

I'll have to get a better-paying job.
What then?
I'll have to go back to school.
What then?
I don't have the money.
What then?
I'll stay at my job or maybe start a business. I don't know.

The point here is that no one knows the future, while the doomsday scenarios we spin in our heads about the consequences of certain choices are largely fantasies that keep us from moving our lives forward. Once we understand this, our doubts and fears lose much of their power.

EXERCISE:
Surrender to the No

The idea behind this exercise is to practice living with the notion that you don't know what's going to happen and that's okay. It's an exercise that's likely to make you feel uncomfortable, which is the whole point. It provides you with the opportunity to practice self-parenting, which means you contain the feelings that arise as a result of putting yourself in an uncomfortable position, process them, and remind yourself that all will be okay. It's about learning to be comfortable with discomfort. The more you practice this, the more you'll be able to move into a state of healthy self-doubt. Try both versions multiple times, and then consider coming up with some ways of your own that allow you to surrender to the "no."

Option 1 Directions

1. Go to a coffee shop or a mall—any safe place of your choosing where you know there will be people.

2. Stand outside for a little while and watch people come and go. Then stop someone and ask that person for money. Any amount is fine.
3. Whatever the person's answer is, whatever the person's reaction is, accept it. A no is as good as a yes.

Option 2 Directions

1. Go to a new safe place where you know there will be people.
2. Stand outside for a little while and watch people come and go. Then stop someone and ask that person for his or her phone number. If the person asks why, say you are looking for a new friend or whatever answer feels right to you.
3. Whatever the person's answer, whatever their reaction is, accept it. Remember, a no is as good as a yes.

The point of these scenarios is to surrender to the outcome before even asking the question. If the answer is no ("No, I won't give you money" or, "There's no way I'm giving you my phone number"), that's fine. You've lost nothing and nothing bad has happened to you. If the answer is yes, then you have a little extra cash to pocket or the potential of a new friend.

This exercise lets you practice sitting with the kind of uncomfortable feelings we so often avoid, such as vulnerability, fear of rejection, lack of control, and embarrassment. Once you've sat with them, guess what happens? It becomes clear there really wasn't anything to fear in the first place. You're okay no matter what the outcome.

A Word about Trust

Embodying healthy self-doubt requires us to trust that everything will be okay. My patient could have trusted that everything would have worked out one way or another if he had only applied for a job on his own merits. You will have to trust that everything is going to be fine if you confront a stranger in the street and ask for money or a phone number. When you worked to uncover buried emotions in the last step, you had to trust that you could handle whatever came up. In a process that requires this level of trust, questions might arise such as *Where am I placing this trust? How can I be so sure everything will work out?*

In moments of unhealthy self-doubt or self-judgment it can help to call on a Higher Power, whatever that means to you. I believe we are each individualized extensions of the one Great Spirit, or God, through which we are all united. The essence of God is love. Since we are an expression of God, love is also our essence. Because the essence of both is love, it means that when we trust that all will work out, what we are trusting in is both this Higher Power and ourselves.

Whether you agree with this or not, you can probably still agree that our experiences make us who we are and have the potential to teach us something. In other words, we can grow as much from our negative experiences as we can from our positive ones. Remember what we talked about in the beginning of this book, how possibilities for positive growth and change are inherent in all problems, even the most difficult ones. Yes, I know we often feel things could be better in our lives, but this doesn't mean we can't benefit from what's happening right now.

This perspective is key to ending the downward spiral of self-criticism, blame, preconceived judgment, and doubt—all the things that keep us stuck. Instead we see ourselves as blameless, innocent souls moving through the maze of life, making choices, experiencing outcomes, and doing it again and again. While the choices we make may not be perfect, we always make the best choices given our level of consciousness at the time. From this perspective there is no such thing as a mistake. There are only choices, outcomes, and the knowledge we gain that will help us improve our choices. When we know better, we make better choices. But knowing better typically involves making a choice that creates a problem in our lives, which we then learn from. This is why there's no need to judge our choices or doubt them, let alone doubt ourselves.

The exercise that follows asks you to practice trusting the universe in the way I've described. I use the term Divine Loving Essence to describe the innocent soul inside each of us whose essence is love. When we see ourselves in this way, we recognize that we are always exactly where we are supposed to be and that everything we are experiencing is for our own growth and highest good. Realizing this will help you move forward in your life with greater clarity.

EXERCISE:
Seeing the Divine Loving Essence in Your Authentic Self

Seeing the Divine Loving Essence in yourself will benefit you in a myriad of ways, including the following:

- Helping to create a loving attitude that supports greater clarity
- Preventing you from being caught in a downward spiral of judgment or self-doubt
- Preventing you from being pulled into unconscious choices.
- Providing you with the opportunity to show yourself the love, compassion, and acceptance you deserve
- Automatically deepening your relationship with your authentic self.

DIRECTIONS

1. Begin by calling in your authentic self in the same way you did for the intention-setting exercise on page 60. As you become

more familiar with the practice over time, you'll be able to call on your authentic self quickly at any time and in any place.

2. As you embody the Divine Loving Essence, remind your judgmental self that good will come out of every situation because, even though you can't see it now, it's all working for your benefit on a higher level. In the most compassionate way, reassure yourself that you always make the best choices given your level of consciousness at the time. Tell that concerned childlike self inside that he or she is blameless and forgiven because there's no such thing as a mistake. There are only choices, outcomes, and the knowledge we gain to make further choices. You can have this conversation internally or out loud. It should be spoken in the voice of the authentic self, the voice that conveys nurturing, protection, and wisdom just like that of a loving parent or friend.

3. If your judgmental self has feedback, hear him or her out and respond from your authentic self. Move between the two aspects of yourself to facilitate a dialogue until trust is established and a sense of peace returns.

This is a great exercise to do whenever you are having a particularly difficult time containing and processing negative emotions such as fear and doubt, or when you're consumed with anger or shame. It takes the focus off these negative ways of thinking and helps you reframe your situation in a more positive, beneficial, and more trusting light.

It can also be a good idea to pull out a picture of yourself as a child when you do this exercise (the younger, the better). Look at the image of the innocent child you once were as you facilitate this loving conversation with yourself. I do something similar with all my patients. I ask them to send me a photo of themselves as a child, which I attach to their contact information in my phone. This way, whenever a patient calls me I see their child self. It's amazing how this automatically opens me up, enhancing my feelings of empathy and affection for them. You're likely to call up similar feelings when you look at a childhood picture of yourself.

Embrace Suffering

Having clarity doesn't mean that we're happy all the time or feel only positive emotions. We saw in an earlier chapter that when we are faced with difficult circumstances, a crucial aspect of creating emotional clarity is to fully feel our feelings, allowing ourselves to grieve such events as the loss of our relationship, loved one, innocence, job, opportunity, or health. It's important to embrace life's ebb and flow. In the context of our psycho-spiritual wellbeing, this means accepting suffering just as we would joy, and doing so without preconceived judgment or resistance.

According to Buddhism there are Four Noble Truths. The first tells us that to live is to suffer. This doesn't mean that all life is suffering, but it does mean that suffering is a natural part of life. Since we can't exist without occasional suffering, perhaps it's time to stop fighting it. To fight expends energy we could be putting to better use by processing our own emotional waste and creating greater clarity. This step aims to help facilitate acceptance of the suffering that's an inevitable part of all our lives.

....

"He who fears he shall suffer, already suffers what he fears."
—Michel de Montaigne

"We are healed of a suffering only by experiencing it to the full."

—Marcel Proust

"Although the world is full of suffering, it is also full of the over-coming of it."

—Helen Keller

"You must submit to supreme suffering in order to discover the completion of joy."

—John Calvin

....

Caesura, or Crisis as Opportunity

Buddha is just one of many wise people throughout history who had something to say about the nature of suffering. Among them is our friend Wilfred Bion, who defined the concept of containment. Bion wrote about another psychological concept called *caesura*, which comes from the Latin meaning "a cut." Our lives, he theorized, are a series of cuts, starting the moment we are born.

We begin our existence by spending nine months in the warm and nurturing environment of our mother's womb, which leads to the violent and traumatic moment of our birth when we come screaming into the world. It's not an easy transition for either mother or baby, but it's a necessary one if we want to continue to live and grow—a basic fact we instinctively accept and understand.

The pattern continues following our birth. When we're hungry we latch on to our mother's breast, until the moment she says no and coaxes us to drink from a bottle and in due course eat solid food. We may cry and resist, but soon we learn how to feed ourselves. These are skills we need to develop if we are to continue to live and grow, which is a basic fact we instinctively accept and understand.

The pattern continues as we navigate milestone after milestone.

Most of us learn to be careful around a hot stove only after we've singed ourselves once or twice. We learn to ride a bicycle by falling off more than once. Eventually we learn enough to be able to leave home and live on our own.

What makes us think this pattern should stop in adulthood? From time to time we may wish there were no more crises, no more difficult or heartbreaking circumstances, but do we really want this? If we didn't experience loss, what would propel us to learn and grow?

Bion's theory of *caesura* suggests that when we are able to contain the experience, any crisis, any cut, becomes an opportunity that forces us to move forward in conscious evolution. Everything I have asked you to do in the second part of this book can be seen as intentional attempts to create small *caesuras*. Consider the cleanse, which asks you to engage in the everyday function of eating in a manner that's new and potentially unwanted. Or think of the PEW 12 exercise, which can bring unhappy feelings to the surface. Then there's the notion that you should sit with your uncomfortable feelings rather than bury or ignore them, as well as the idea that you should embrace suffering. All of these are ways of poking you in different places to see where your pain points lie so you can discover what causes you to emotionally or spiritually cry *Ouch*.

I often tell my patients, "I can't be your mentor if you won't let me be your tormentor." I once had a patient in the ER who yelled out and instinctively took a swing at me when I pressed on his abdomen. He was furious with me because of the pain I'd caused him, until I explained how this one moment of pain, sharp as it was, probably saved his life. It was the clue I needed to diagnose his appendicitis and send him for emergency surgery. The same would happen were I to press on your wrist. If the bone is in good shape, you wouldn't mind the extra pressure. Only if your wrist is fractured would you feel pain and cry out.

Like a diagnostician's hands or an acupuncturist's needle, we're searching for the blockages of energy inside ourselves. It's not an easy or comfortable process, but it's necessary for finding out where our internal fractures lie. The primary thing to keep in mind is that the pain won't kill you. The secondary point is that each of these moments is an opportunity to practice being okay with pain and suffering so that we can move forward and grow from the experience.

All too often we miss these opportunities. We're too busy avoiding or repressing the negative feelings that arise from unwanted experiences to take the time to explore the lessons they have to teach us. Our basic instinct tells us to either ignore or run from suffering for the simple reason it feels bad. But keep in mind that when we choose *not* to ignore or run from it, we give ourselves the chance to fully feel our feelings so that the negative energy doesn't build up inside us.

If through denial or avoidance we refuse to suffer emotionally, we will suffer in other ways, such as by continuing to make the same mistakes over and over again, feeling unfulfilled or disempowered, or even suffering physically (as we've seen with many of the patients whose stories I've told thus far). In contrast, to suffer the emotional pain of a negative experience as it's happening is to honor our experiences. It's also what will allow us to give meaning to those experiences, as we shall see shortly.

Suffering allows us to keep the momentum of our lives moving. As we work through the catabolic or breaking-down phases of our lives that suffering inspires, we can use what we learn from our difficult circumstances to build our lives back up so that they are better, and we are better, than before our problems occurred. This is how our lives evolve, how we evolve as people.

Letting Your Suffering Lead You Inward

The notion that suffering should be embraced as an opportunity to learn and grow requires a shift in consciousness. With this in mind, let me suggest a way of looking at this that might make the shift easier to digest.

We've been mistakenly taught to fear the dark, whereas in truth the dark is a gift. If the light in the room you're sitting in right now were to suddenly go out so that you were left in total darkness, you'd almost surely be frightened. However, as I related when my wife took me to the restaurant where we ate in the dark, all your non-visual senses would become more acute in order to compensate for your lack of vision. This is why people who are blind so often have a heightened sense of hearing. The darkness makes us more conscious of things we mostly ignore in our usual state of awareness. In other words, the darkness doesn't hide things but reveals them.

When we close our eyes, our brainwave activity immediately begins to decrease. We leave the normal waking beta frequency of 13 to 30 cycles per second (Hz) and enter the alpha range of 8 to 12 Hz. At this frequency parts of our brain that are usually busy processing billions of bits of visual data each second become freed up, making them available to process information from a completely different source. The darkness of the alpha range is where our creative mind becomes engaged, inspiration is born, and answers are received. In Sanskrit, the word *nirvana* actually means "to blow out," as in to blow out a candle. The word seems to signal the idea that our personal paradise can be found not in the bright world around us, but in the still, quiet darkness within.

What is suffering if not the dark night of our soul? When we go into the darkness as a result of suffering, it will always lead us back to the light. The winter solstice, which is the shortest and thus darkest day of the year, is also a turning point. Once the solstice is over, the days grow longer and more filled with light. The dark night of our soul is no different, so let's befriend it. This is the thought that I want you to hold in your mind as you use the exercises that follow to help you embrace your suffering. After all, the dark night of our soul is a signal that the light is coming. It has the potential to reveal to you your nirvana.

EXERCISE:
Tide Breathing, or Breathing through the Sadness

Embracing suffering is one of those quintessential *easier-said-than-done* situations. It's hard to do because it involves doing nothing.

A few years ago my beloved brother, to whom I've dedicated this book, passed away far too young. While I was mourning his passing, I took ten days off and went to Cancún, which I chose because it was near the location where he and I last scuba-dived together. Although I reserved a room at the beach, I hardly ever came out of it. Instead I left the balcony door wide open, allowing myself to be in sync with the rhythm of the tide. Then I just breathed my suffering out and into the ocean.

Breathing is a powerful tool because it creates space. Your lungs literally expand inside you, opening up space within and filling it with air. If you can breathe through your suffering, you can tolerate it. That's what this next exercise will teach you:

1. Find somewhere you can sit quietly. Close your eyes and sit in darkness for a moment. As you do, make sure not to hold your breath, but continue to let your breath flow in and out.
2. Next picture the ocean. It has a rhythm. Notice the rhythm that's created by the flow of water coming in, then rushing out, coming in, then rushing out. Once you get a sense of the ocean's rhythm, let your breath follow it. Inhale as the water comes in, exhale as it recedes, inhale as the water comes in, exhale as it recedes, and on and on.

3. After a while you'll notice that you've begun to breathe more deeply. When this happens, allow your breath to have a voice as it flows out of you—a kind of *ahhhhhhhhh*. The sound will carry with it some of the tension you are holding.

4. Continue with this until your body relaxes and your mind calms. Each time you breathe through your sorrow rather than retreat from it, it will reinforce for you the truth that it isn't going to kill you. You can bear more than you think.

EXERCISE:
Prizing, or Refocusing Your Negative Energy

When we're suffering it can seem there's no way out. We may even feel like giving up on trying to improve our situation. In such a situation, prizing—which means to value highly—is a powerful tool we can use to redirect our energy away from feeling sad, angry, or hopeless about our situation. By prizing—or *praising*—ourselves, we allow ourselves to truly see and feel the Divine Loving Essence within. Verbalizing the truth of what we see and feel enables us to switch our focus from the problem to the possibilities.

We have all the resources and wisdom we need inside of us to weather any situation we may face and come out on the other side better for the experience. By focusing on the qualities embodied in our authentic self—such as courage, strength, resourcefulness, intelligence, and creativity—we reinforce our ability to draw on these qualities to resolve any difficult or painful situation we find ourselves in. Prizing is an opportunity for us to demonstrate our deeply felt self-love. We acknowledge to ourselves, *"I am a beautiful, bright soul, doing the best I can given the givens!"*

Things to Remember

Prizing yourself in times of suffering

- allows you to take your power back and achieve a sense of peace and control over the situation
- improves your self-esteem by acknowledging and praising all you've done to help yourself
- recognizes and reinforces your awareness of your own Divine Loving Essence through compassion, encouragement, and self-appreciation
- inspires new ideas that may contribute to resolving the situation or issue.

DIRECTIONS:

1. Once again, begin by calling in your authentic self in the same way you did for the intention-setting exercise on page 60.
2. When you feel centered in your authentic self, ask your judgmental self why it's feeling scared, hopeless, frustrated, or stuck.
3. Answer this question from the perspective of your judgmental self, allowing all your emotions to come to the fore. Let your judgmental self discharge as much negative energy as it needs to.
4. When you've finished, reply to the same question you formed in number two from the consciousness of your authentic self, using positive and encouraging words. This is an opportunity to soothe the judgmental self, to let it know that it has been heard, then to bring a more positive perspective to the situation. Your reply might sound something like this:

Your loss of a big client today was a setback that understandably has left you feeling down, but this doesn't make you a failure. You're an excellent businessman with a deep knowledge of this industry. Your courage and insight grew this company from its meager beginnings, and it's those same qualities that will see it recover and thrive following this loss. You are a leader.

Betrayal is painful, and you've been so brave through all of this, especially for your children. The dignified way in which you've conducted yourself proves you're committed to saving your marriage. Even if it doesn't work out, you have all the intelligence, resourcefulness, and creativity you need to build a wonderful and fulfilling new life for yourself and your children.

I can see how difficult it has been for you, and it's a testament to your strength and maturity that you've chosen to act in a professional manner when your boss tries to sabotage you. You are an expert in your field and an exemplary employee. Your record speaks for itself. Regardless of what happens at work, you'll be a highly desirable asset to any firm. Do you remember how many calls you got the last time you sent out résumés?

Let Go of the "Why Me"

When you are able to embrace your suffering, you can establish a relationship with your disease, divorce, unhappiness, or other issue. From this position there's nothing adversarial about your attitude, nothing to fight, no wishing things were different. This doesn't mean you don't take the necessary steps to support yourself. You may still undergo surgery to cut out a cancerous tumor, engage a lawyer to represent you in your divorce, or go back to school so you can prepare yourself for a new and more fulfilling career. But whatever steps you take, you take them without regret or self-judgment.

So far we've covered how life is a series of cuts. We've seen that we should be curious about negative events and how they make us feel. We've also discussed the importance of asking open-ended questions such as *Why am I feeling this way?* or *What can I learn from this traumatic experience?* These are worthwhile perspectives and help us to ask further worthwhile questions. However, some open-ended questions, like *Why me?* or *Why am I suffering?* aren't helpful. We can stop asking ourselves these questions because the answer is always the same. We suffer because all creatures suffer. It's just a part of life.

While suffering often inspires feelings of sadness, it can also inspire anger, which is the birthplace of the question *Why me?* People often object "I don't deserve this, so why is it happening to me?"

"Why me? I don't understand it" was one of the first things that Anne, a 42-year-old real estate agent with breast cancer, said to me during our first appointment. "I eat all organic food and have practiced transcendental meditation for over 20 years. How does someone like me get cancer? This wasn't supposed to happen." She felt betrayed by the world. How could someone who had done all the "right things" end up with cancer at such a young age?

The first point I shared with her was that, while her diet would be an important aspect of her healing, it was only *a part* of the process. No matter how healthy our habits are, our health isn't primarily derived from what we eat but from what we digest. Based on my personal experience with hundreds of patients, the real healing shift comes not when patients change their lifestyle but when they find the emotional component that's supporting their disease, then do the necessary psycho-spiritual work to release it.

Anger, as it turned out, was a big part of Anne's life, particularly anger at men. She was married, but she wasn't shy about expressing her negative opinion of her husband—or, for that matter, of practically any man she talked about. For me this was a clue to which pain points I needed to press. Sure enough, through our work together, I discovered that Anne had been traumatized during her childhood by an enraged father who abused her mother in front of her.

Anne admitted that this experience led her to resent and mistrust men in her adult life. Eventually she had married although she had only engaged in sex with her husband a handful of times, and even then it was mostly because she wanted a child. Two months after she gave birth to her daughter, she noticed that when her husband returned from an out-of-town bachelor party, he was acting distant. The situation escalated until her husband finally confessed he'd had a one-night fling. Of course, this confirmed all of Anne's negative perceptions about men, and things went from bad to worse in her marriage.

Considering Anne's general beliefs about men, I was surprised she didn't leave her husband immediately. Instead she chose to stay with him because she wanted a second child. The baby came, but nothing else changed except that Anne was diagnosed with breast cancer a couple of years later.

I have found that anger and resentment are among the most common emotional attachments related to cancer. Anne's years of resentment toward her father, her husband, and men in general were the cancer that was eating away at her. I suspect she only trusted me, a male doctor, because I was recommended to her by a female friend I had successfully treated. As caustic as she came across when she spoke about men, I had little doubt she felt powerless around them and that her inability to assert herself was keeping her stuck.

Anne eventually made the decision to have a mastectomy, but without radiation or chemotherapy. I stressed to her that unless she did the proper work and dissolved her emotional saturation of anger and resentment, there was no guarantee her cancer wouldn't return. To her credit she got to work, in particular by creating authentic communication with her husband and then her father, whom she hadn't spoken to since college. It was difficult for her to open up to these men whom she'd had such negative feelings about for so long, but she didn't let herself quit. She was determined to heal in as many ways as she could—her relationships, her spirit, her body. It was a long road, but she recently celebrated her 17th wedding anniversary. She now even boasts about having sex three times a week! She's also had her father over for dinner several times and they have come to understand each other better. Best of all, she remains cancer-free.

Anne's story is a powerful example of the idea that we don't have to love our problem, but we do have to acknowledge that it's here to help us. From this perspective we can begin a dialogue with it, which will allow us to heal and ultimately grow.

Give Meaning to Suffering

Although suffering is an unavoidable fact of life, this doesn't mean that life is all about suffering. We embrace suffering in order to learn from it, not to live a life filled with little else. Once we've taken what we can use from the experience of suffering, the next step is to move past it. We do this by giving meaning to our suffering.

When we consciously assign meaning to something, we take responsibility for shaping our lives. Yes, bad things happen, and often those things are beyond our control. But as the Greek philosopher Epictetus once wrote, "It's not what happens to you but how you react to it that matters." In every situation, each of us gets to decide for ourselves how we will react to what happens to us and what meaning we will attach to these events. How we choose to define the events and people in our lives will determine how we ultimately define ourselves. In short, the meaning we choose to give to things matters a great deal, not just with respect to whatever may be causing our suffering but to our entire lives, including our very sense of self.

Yet all too often we leave meaning up to chance. Something happens to us that makes us feel bad or good, and without thinking too much about it we internalize our reaction. Once internalized, it guides our actions, reactions, thoughts, and feelings going forward, even if it was based on a misperception or overreaction.

A patient of mine I'll call Gina told me a story about being bullied years before when she was in high school. While attending a summer party with her boyfriend, the two of them decided to go upstairs to have sex. Because she was obviously focused on their activity, she didn't notice at first when a young man entered the room holding a video camera. At some point his movement caught the corner of her eye. When she sat up to see who was there, she inadvertently provided the camera with a clear shot of her breasts.

Gina and her boyfriend yelled at the intruder to get out, which he did. Unfortunately they didn't think to get the tape from him. Without Gina's knowledge, the boy distributed copies of the video to practically all of the kids in their community. Gina only discovered what he had done on her first day of school, after she had been called a slut so many times she lost count.

This kind of school bullying is often traumatizing because children haven't yet developed their full capacity to process their emotions and assign their own meaning to things, particularly to something so painful. Since everyone had concluded that Gina was a slut, in her young mind she decided this meant she really was a slut. She felt alone and ashamed. To compensate, she said she'd do practically anything to be liked. This included having sex with lots of boys at her school.

I didn't meet Gina until she was in her 30s, by which point the idea that she was a slut had affected her relationships, her sense of self, and her health for years. We worked together to release the emotions related to her trauma, subjugation, and humiliation, assigning new meaning to the events she had experienced. Only after she was able to see herself as a person worthy of love and acceptance could the suffering resulting from her high school trauma truly end.

What Does Meaning *Mean?*

In this step you are going to learn how to consciously assign meaning to any event, particularly the negative or difficult ones, in ways that will move you forward rather than leave you mired in suffering. But first let's look more closely at what I mean when I talk about giving *meaning* to something. To illustrate this concept, consider the following medieval tale:

A traveler came to a work site and saw two men carrying stones. One man was working listlessly, with a sullen expression on his face, while the other was cheerfully singing as he busily carried stone after stone.

"What are you doing?" the traveler asked the sullen worker.

"Laying stone," the worker replied.

"What are you doing?" asked the traveler of the industrious worker.

"Building a cathedral," he replied.

This simple story illustrates how two people can assign a very different meaning to the same circumstances. Given the crucial difference between "I have to work" versus "I am being of service," which of these two workers would you rather be?

Another way to define what we're doing is to give something context. An example comes from the book *On Being Certain* by Robert A. Burton, MD:

A newspaper is better than a magazine. A seashore is a better place than a street. At first it is better to run than to walk. You may have to try several times. It takes some skill, but it is easy to learn. Even young children can enjoy it. Once successful, complications are minimal. Birds seldom get too close. Rain, however, soaks in very fast. Too many people doing the same thing can also cause problems. One needs lots of room. If there are no complications it can be very peaceful. A rock will serve as an anchor. If things break loose from it, however, you will not get a second chance.

Now read the passage again, only this time it has been given a title.

Kite

A newspaper is better than a magazine. A seashore is a better place than a street. At first it is better to run than to walk. You may have to try several times. It takes some skill, but it is easy to learn. Even young children can enjoy it. Once successful, complications are minimal. Birds seldom get too close. Rain, however, soaks in very fast. Too many people doing the same thing can also cause problems. One needs lots of room. If there are no complications it can be very peaceful. A rock will serve as an anchor. If things break loose from it, however, you will not get a second chance.

What's the difference between these two passages? Just one word, *kite*, which serves as the title of the second passage. Yet this one word makes all the difference. The title, made up of just four letters, is what gives the passage context because it imparts meaning. Without it all you have is a jumble of seemingly random thoughts and words. It's nonsense. But with a title in place, the ideas in the passage suddenly make sense.

Our thoughts and feelings about the things that happen to us, particularly those that cause us to suffer, are a bit like this passage when it's read without a title. They can be elusive, hard to understand, confusing, and possibly misleading. Similarly, emotions we can't make sense of can end up guiding us, as they did with Gina, instead of us guiding them. This is why it's so important we learn how to contain them.

Recall the metaphor of the cup and Wilfred Bion's theory of containment. We want to hold feelings that don't make sense to us and sit with our reaction long enough for us to identify and understand what we are experiencing. Only then can we decide what these feelings mean to us.

The order is important here. If we don't process our emotions first, we risk assigning meaning based on misinterpretations, misidentifications, misperceptions, and misunderstandings. We also leave ourselves open to external pressures, relying on what other people think or what society tells us something means rather than deciding for ourselves. This isn't an empowering way to give our lives meaning.

I find a problem with many approaches to psycho-spiritual healing today, in that they too often ignore the processing and skip straight to assigning meaning to experiences. They talk about the power of positive thinking or tuning into self-love without providing a framework for how to do so, rendering such advice little more than wishful thinking. You could force yourself to think positively about the jumble of ideas in the first passage quoted above, but what good would it do you if you hadn't taken the time to understand it? By the same token, you could force yourself to adopt a positive view of your circumstances. But if you haven't given yourself the time and space to understand them and how you got into them, how does your positive thinking really serve you? Perhaps more importantly, how long do you think that positivity will last?

The title "Kite" gives functionality to the passage. When we access the functionality of an experience, we give it meaning. In order to do this, we have to be able to look at the situation from an elevated perspective, a kind of bird's-eye point of view, which allows us to see it clearly in its entirety and put it in a new context. We can't do this if we're mired in the muck of our uncontained emotions.

Meaning Versus Judgment

Humans' conception of the world has altered as our perspective has evolved. Early humans believed the oceans or mountains that limited their travel delineated the very edge of the world itself. For generations, people believed the earth was flat, until ships were able to carry them across oceans and they discovered they didn't fall off the edge.

Our perspective expanded even further when we were able to see the earth from an airplane. When we finally viewed the planet from space, this elevated perspective changed the entire context of our world. We no longer had to imagine how the earth looks because we could actually see images that revealed its round shape, free of edges or sides. The idea that anything has sides in a singular universe based on wholeness and balance is an illusion.

Judgment is about taking sides. Anytime emotional upset is uncontained, we judge what happened to us as bad based on how it makes us feel. Next we judge the people and circumstances involved, and especially ourselves. Judgments like *I'm unlovable, I'm helpless, I'm a victim, It's my fault, It's his fault, It's her fault* saturate our consciousness. We quickly learn *good* things always feel good and are to be pursued, while *bad* things are to be avoided, feared, or resisted.

Out of context (remember the kite passage), anything can be "bad." For example, when we're thirsty we might reach for water to drink. As long as water is pure, we generally think of water as a good thing. But is it always? If we drink too much of it, even water can become a toxin. You may recall seeing news reports of fraternity hazing rituals getting out of hand when individuals pledged to drink gallons and gallons of water, only to end up in hospital or dying from water intoxication or *hyponatremia*. Nothing, not even water, is inherently good or bad. When we view things as if they were inherently good or bad, seeing them in a polarized way, we are coming from a place of judgment and misunderstanding.

Instead of judging or taking sides when something difficult happens in our lives, we can integrate the experience. We can take it in so that we understand it, process it, then take what we can use to move our lives forward. We can make any experience useful, viewed as something to learn and grow from, no matter how difficult or painful it is. We do this by assigning new meaning to it instead of judging it as good or bad, right or wrong. We can't create clarity unless we can understand this crucial insight.

My patient Raffi struggled with this distinction when he hit a crisis point in his life. I had known Raffi for several years when he called me one day out of the blue in a frantic state. He had just arrived home from a business trip to find his belongings packed and left for him in the foyer. He wandered from room to room, looking for someone to provide him with an explanation, but neither his wife nor any of their four children were anywhere to be found. As he searched the house, he noticed that every single photo of him had been removed as if someone was trying to erase him from his own life.

Unsure what to do, Raffi gathered his things and went to a hotel for the night. When he returned home the next day, the locks had been changed. Calls to his wife and children went unanswered and unreturned. He soon discovered that even his bank accounts had been frozen. When he left for the business trip a week earlier, he thought everything was fine. Upon his return, he discovered that his entire life had been turned upside down.

In the following days and weeks, I talked regularly with Raffi. I'd never witnessed anyone so consumed with anxiety, depression, rage, and confusion. When I asked him why he thought his wife had done this, he was so saturated with emotion that all he could do was point the finger at her. "She did this to me," he raged. "It's all *her* fault." Meanwhile his wife would only communicate with him through her lawyer, which meant Raffi was unable to talk with her about why she had taken such extreme action. His feelings of blame and hatred for her intensified to the point he was eventually admitted to hospital with an ulcer that was causing him to violently vomit blood. It was only after this scare that he was able to take a step back and focus not on blaming his wife but on his own emotional healing.

As it turned out, Raffi had a lot of ground to cover, going back to early childhood when his mother left his father without warning. The move had rendered his father so heartbroken that he abandoned Raffi, taking off and living out the rest of his days by himself. A few years later, the father died of what Raffi always assumed was a broken heart.

As Raffi continued to focus on himself, he realized he had never gotten past what his mother and father had done all those years earlier. Holding on to that resentment and pain had caused him to grow into an emotionally unavailable adult who kept his wife and children at arm's length. This, he imagined, was the primary factor that drove his wife away, an insight she confirmed for him when, two weeks before their divorce hearing, she finally agreed to meet him for lunch. It was the first direct contact they'd had with each other in months, and it turned out to be the most candid and emotionally open conversation they had ever had with each other. During the course of the conversation, they were both brought to tears over the ending of their 25 years together. While his wife still felt she needed to terminate the marriage and move on, she agreed to arbitration instead of going through with what could have been a protracted battle in the courts.

The shift Raffi made as a result of the work we did together was the same shift we all have to make, moving from judgment to love. Raffi shifted from blaming his wife for tearing his life apart to thanking her for opening his eyes to what was missing in his life. Assigning this new meaning to his heart-wrenching circumstances allowed him to move past his anger and work on loving himself. It was a difficult journey, but he would say that it was more than worth the effort. Today he has a loving, healthy relationship with all his children and makes it a priority to spend time with them and his grandchildren. He's even friendly with his ex-wife. Most of all, he understands the gift he was given through his suffering, because without it he wouldn't have learned how much joy there is in feeling emotionally connected to those closest to him.

....

Out beyond ideas of wrongdoing and rightdoing,
there is a field. I'll meet you there.
When the soul lies down in that grass,
the world is too full to talk about.
Ideas, language, even the phrase each other
doesn't make any sense.

—Rumi, 13th century, translated by Coleman
Barks in *The Essential Rumi*

....

There's Judgment and Then There's Judgment

In much the same way that there is healthy self-doubt and unhealthy self-doubt, there are two kinds of judgment—one that can help us navigate our lives, the other that will limit our possibilities and keep us stuck.

Let's talk about the limiting kind first, which I generally refer to as *preconceived judgments*. These types of judgments are based on past experiences rather than a full understanding and processing of the situation unfolding before us.

Suppose you're hiking through the mountains one day and encounter a snake. In that moment, your mind may go back to a time in school when you learned about rattlesnakes and the poisonous venom they employ against their enemies. Or maybe you recall a story from the Bible, where it was a snake's crafty and duplicitous nature that led to Adam and Eve being cast out of the Garden of Eden. You may even have had an encounter with a poisonous snake, and this is what you call up at this moment. Whatever the case, that past experience dovetails in your mind with your present circumstances, causing you to say to yourself, "That's a snake! I'm in danger! I must run."

Most of the time this kind of thought process happens unconsciously. But what if the snake you've encountered is simply a run-of-the-mill garden snake? It has no venom and no other ability to harm. Despite the snap judgment telling you to run, you're in no danger. Of course, there's probably no harm in running from a garden snake, but there can be real harm as a result of other kinds of preconceived judgments. For example, after Raffi's parents abandoned him, deep down he judged himself unworthy of love. As an adult he brought this judgment against himself into his marriage, where it kept him from achieving closeness and intimacy with his wife.

Not all judgments limit or hold us back. In fact we need to be able to make *conscious judgments* in order to move our lives forward. For example, if we own a business, we may need to hire people to help us. To do this we might post an ad and receive a variety of résumés in response. We have to be able to look at these résumés and judge who would be best suited for the position based on his or her experience and character. The trick is to base this judgment on the information we have in front of us rather than on some preconceived idea about how a certain type of person might perform. After all, another name for preconceived judgments could be bias or prejudice.

When we allow ourselves to make conscious judgments rather

than reacting to our preconceived ones, we give ourselves the gift of choice. The answer to what we will do in any given situation isn't predetermined by a past experience. We get to choose whether to look more closely at that garden snake or let it be. We get to choose who we wish to work with on a daily basis.

Once Raffi was able to look at the events that led up to his wife leaving him with fresh eyes, he still had some choices to make about his life and how best to move forward. For instance, he and his wife needed to decide what sort of arrangement would work for their children. By employing their conscious judgment to make these kinds of decisions, they were able to make choices that served the greatest good for all concerned.

People often throw around the word *judgment* as if it's a bad thing. We call someone "judgmental" when we want to accuse him or her of treating us wrongly or unfairly. However, as we make our way toward greater clarity, we will be best served if we remember that judgment isn't inherently right or wrong, good or bad. There are judgments that limit us and there are judgments that help us move our lives forward. Our job is to try to catch ourselves when we gravitate toward the first kind and instead move toward making more conscious judgments whenever possible.

Reframing Events

Letting go of our preconceived judgments and, in their place, choosing to give new meaning to something is an act of reframing or recontextualizing. When we learn how to reframe illness, tragedy, or suffering as a means to a positive end, we can transform our entire experience. We can create a new energy in our lives, one that supports our psycho-spiritual and physical healing, thus expanding our world.

This isn't an exercise in putting lipstick on a pig or looking through rose-colored glasses. The goal isn't merely to attain a more positive view of our circumstances, but to come to a more real and truthful view.

Think about Gina. Because of an unfortunate event that happened when she was still young, her classmates judged her as a slut worthy of little more than ridicule. As a result she held that same judgment against herself long after the event was over and she'd left the community where it occurred. I contend that nothing about this judgment was real or true. Instead it was a cruel and unnecessary interpretation of what happened, which kept part of her from growing and moving forward with her life for a long time.

When we internalize the idea that we are a lost cause, somehow broken beyond repair, it not only impacts us at the time we make this assessment, it can remain with us and influence our future beliefs and behavior for years.

A Japanese pottery technique called kintsukuroi perfectly explains how brokenness is really an illusion. In the 15th century, Japanese shogun Ashikaga Yoshimasa sent a precious but damaged Chinese tea bowl back to China for repairs. Disappointed when it came back to him with crude metal bindings holding the pieces together, he employed craftsmen of his own to find a more aesthetically pleasing solution. The metal clasps were removed and the pottery shards set in place using a lacquer resin. To hide the adhesive and add elegance to the bowl's appearance, the craftsmen sprinkled powdered gold over the seams of the repair. The end result was a piece that was more beautiful than it had been before it was broken. In fact what started as a repair for broken pottery quickly became an artisan technique that was much sought after in Japan. Kintsukuroi actually translates as *golden repair* or *to repair with gold*. Since then ceramics have often been broken intentionally so this technique can be applied for the purpose of creating great beauty.

How might our lives be different if we chose to see ourselves not as broken down by our suffering, but rather in the process of a repair from which we'll emerge as something far more beautiful than when we began? After all, things of great beauty rarely appear out of nowhere. A great sculptor doesn't simply wish upon a star when creating an exquisite figure of an angel. He takes a blunt block of marble and works it, chipping away, removing pieces, smoothing edges, until the figure inside finally emerges. A diamond begins as a crude, dull crystal and must face weeks at the grinding wheel before it becomes the brilliant scintillation that dazzles us.

As you work on giving meaning to your suffering, it's important to remember that although it may feel like everything is breaking down, this isn't the same as being broken. Remember, breaking down or catabolism is a natural phase of life. You may be breaking down, but you're not missing any of your parts. You haven't lost anything that's essential to who you are or what you need in order to heal. You're still complete and can never be otherwise. You simply require a rearrangement of pieces from time to time, a reframing of ideas in order to see things in a new way.

The following exercises will help you work through rearranging the pieces of your life, reframing your suffering, and choosing to see things in a new way in order to leave you and your life more beautiful as a result of your experiences.

EXERCISE:
The ~~Confession~~ Revelation Booth—Part One

No one gets to think your thoughts but you, which means you are fully in charge and responsible for deciding what meaning will be attached to every person, every event, every single thing that has touched your life. The following exercise is based on the idea of the confession booth used in the Catholic religion. It will help you reframe anything that has caused you suffering or discomfort, allowing you to move from limiting judgment to a meaning focused on growth, expansion, and love. Then in the next step we'll complete the exercise through an act of forgiveness just like you would receive from a priest who took your confession.

DIRECTIONS

1. Take a piece of paper and divide it down the middle lengthwise. On the top of the left-hand column write, "Judgment." On the top of the right-hand column write, "Loving Meaning."
2. At the top of the page write down a brief description of whatever the issue is that you're currently suffering from or struggling with.

<u>Examples:</u> Raffi might have written this:

My wife has left me and separated me from my children.

Gina might have written this:

My privacy has been violated and my classmates are bullying me as a result.

3. Next focus on the judgment column. Write down a list of any judgments you can think of about what happened.

<u>Examples:</u> Raffi might have written these:

My wife is a bitch.
This is all her fault.
My children are ungrateful.

Maybe this is my fault.
Maybe I drove them away.
They're better off without me.
I don't deserve their love.

Gina might have written these:

That boy who took that video is an evil jerk.
This is all his fault.
I'm so embarrassed I can't face anyone.
Everyone hates me because they think I'm a slut.
I must be a slut if everyone says so.
No one will like me if I don't give them what they want.
No one will ever respect me.
I'm not worthy of their respect anyway.

4. Look at each judgment and, one by one, think about how you
   could assign a new meaning to it. Before you do, you may want
   to call on your authentic self and/or go back to the Divine
   Loving Essence exercise in step six. These exercises may help
   you reframe your judgments in a more empowering, truthful,
   and loving way. You might also think about the idea that, as
   you do this, you are applying love to the places inside you that
   are hurting. This is how healing will happen.

Examples: Raffi might have written this:

Limiting Judgment	Loving Meaning
My wife is a bitch.	My wife is still the same strong and passionate woman I fell in love with. I may not know exactly why she left me, but I do know that it was for the highest good of all concerned—for her, for our children, and even for me.

This is all her fault.	She has given me an opportunity to better understand the barriers that are keeping me from feeling fully loved by and connected to those closest to me. I thank her for this gift even if it wasn't her intention to help me in this way.

Gina might have written this:

Limiting Judgment	*Loving Meaning*
I'm so embarrassed I can't face anyone.	I may have put myself in a vulnerable position, but I didn't know what would happen. I wasn't doing anything wrong, but I can still learn something from this. I can learn how to consciously avoid putting myself in a position where people can take advantage of me in the future.
I must be a slut if everyone says so.	I have learned that other people don't define who I am. Only I can do that, and I know I am a beautiful, strong, and loving person who is worthy of love and acceptance even if that's not what I'm feeling right now.

5. After you've written down your new meanings in the right-hand column, consider the following questions:
   - What belief about myself could this person or event be revealing to me?
   - Have I been shown this belief before in other circumstances?
   - If so, why didn't I react appropriately when I received those messages?
   - This person or event provided this experience so my life could be changed for the better in what way?
   - What experiences have I had since the incident that verify this improvement?
   - In what way has this person or event been my teacher?

EXERCISE:
Rewrite Your Memoir

This exercise can be particularly meaningful for anyone who is suffering from old wounds, especially ones that date back to childhood. The word *memoir* comes from the French *mémoire*, which means memory or reminiscence. A person who writes their memoir looks back over the events of their life and records their personal memories of what happened. Many of our early traumas get internalized as narratives or stories we tell ourselves about what happened to us and why we are the way we are. In this exercise, we're going to rewrite those narratives the way we want them to play out now, bringing compassion and love to what has occurred in our past. We're not going to pretend we didn't suffer, but we're going to write a new context for that suffering.

DIRECTIONS

1. Take a notebook and a pen and sit down in a quiet place where you won't be disturbed. Think about a traumatic moment from your past that you want to create a new relationship with. Review the details of that narrative in your mind.
2. Before you begin writing, you may want to call in your authentic self in the same way you did on page 60. You may also want to review the questions in step five of the previous exercise to help you think about this event in a new way (p. 162).
3. Rewrite the story of what happened to you, focusing on how you want it to turn out in the end. With each word, try to bring compassion and love to the person you were back then and to the events you were experiencing. Write from a place of expansion, not contraction. Let yourself feel the suffering, but don't

dwell on that suffering. Give meaning to your suffering by appreciating how it has taught or transformed you, then allow yourself to move forward.

Example: Gina might rewrite the story of her high school trauma this way:

When I was just a teenager, I chose to act passionately at a party. I put myself in a vulnerable position. I don't blame myself. I was young and still learning how to make choices that would better serve me. I had a lot to learn in that area, but I did the best I could with what I knew.

The way others responded to me during that period in my life was very difficult. I felt hurt by this. I acted on this hurt in ways that didn't serve me. But I also learned a lot about how strong and resilient I am. I was just a child, so vulnerable and so alone. Even so, I weathered those hard times and went on to create a beautiful life for myself. I have a wonderful husband and daughter. I'm a physical therapist who gets to help people through their difficulties on a daily basis. I wouldn't be as good at my job, and wouldn't be as good a wife and mother as I am now, if I didn't know what it's like to suffer, as well as what it's like to overcome suffering. My experiences have given me a compassion and empathy for people that I can use to deepen all the relationships in my life, professional and personal. This is my story, and I embrace it fully and hold it in the light.

Helpful Hint: As you write your memoir with new meaning, it may be helpful to picture yourself far into the future looking back on yourself and what you're feeling in this moment. I did this recently, picturing myself on my deathbed on a specific date, April 1, 2070, which will be the day before my 100th birthday. I began by picturing what I might look and sound like. Then I had a dialogue between the two versions of myself. My future self was able to contextualize and reframe for me many of the situations I felt angry about or hurt by, showing much compassion and wisdom in the process. Thinking about my judgments from this perspective created a kind of space within me that allowed me to see things with clearer eyes and a more open heart.

Searching for Meaning

Viktor Frankl was a psychiatrist, neurologist, and Holocaust survivor whose memoir *Man's Search for Meaning*, about his time in a Nazi concentration camp, can serve as inspiration for anyone on a similar quest to find meaning in their own lives. Frankl went on to develop logotherapy, which is based on the idea that meaning is the most powerful driving force in any person's life. (*Logos* comes from a Greek word that can be translated as "meaning.") When thinking about reframing the most difficult events in your life, consider that Frankl was able to do so in the harshest of circumstances for the sake of his own spiritual survival. His book has inspired millions of people and I highly recommend it. In the meantime, here are some words of wisdom from Frankl that are likely to help you through this step.

> Ultimately, man should not ask what the meaning of his life is, but rather must recognize that it is he who is asked. In a word, each man is questioned by life; and he can only answer to life by answering for his own life; to life he can only respond by being responsible.
>
> In some ways suffering ceases to be suffering at the moment it finds a meaning, such as the meaning of a sacrifice.
>
> I do not forget any good deed done to me & I do not carry a grudge for a bad one.

Forgive

Forgiveness is tricky. Things we forgive too quickly don't stay forgiven. Things we refuse to forgive build up and pollute us internally. Despite the fact that forgiveness is challenging, it's essential. It completes the cycle of suffering, processing feelings, deciding what meaning to give to our experiences, and finally letting go. That release can only happen through forgiveness.

After a trauma or difficult experience, forgiveness is what gets us moving again. Without it we become stuck. Remember the septic system? When the system isn't flowing properly and it slows or backs up, problems start. If the blockage isn't removed, things will degenerate over time, contaminating the environment and eventually causing the entire system to break down.

By neutralizing resentful thoughts and feelings, forgiveness serves as the antidote to this kind of breakdown. Rather than giving us a temporary reprieve from blame and judgment, it removes them from our internal environment. When we forgive someone (which often needs to be ourselves), we release any grudges we hold against a person, together with the negative charge connected to the situation. Free of that burden, we move forward with clarity.

Forgiveness can be especially difficult when someone has committed a serious offense against us. However, the biggest mistake most make is to assume that forgiveness is for the benefit of the other. In fact forgiveness has nothing to do with the other person and everything to do with the one doing the forgiving. Forgiveness doesn't let the other off the hook, doesn't grant absolution to the perpetrator. It grants freedom to ourselves so we can flourish.

This common misconception is perhaps the biggest and most difficult hurdle to overcome when forgiving someone. As difficult as it may be, it's a crucial step that can't be skipped. No matter what has happened to us, as long as we view ourselves as "victims" we will not heal. In order to be a victim, there has to be a bad guy who did something to us. Good and bad are opposites that create polarity and judgment, right versus wrong. When there are two opposing sides to anything, resistance is created. When there is resistant energy in the body, healing energy can't flow. We need to learn to forgive for our own sake.

This step is going to help you make your way to forgiveness, whether the person you need to forgive is a stranger, someone close to you, or even—and perhaps especially—yourself.

Courage

The word *courage* comes from the Latin word *cor* and the French *coeur*, both of which mean "heart." The heart was once believed to be the seat of all emotions, including and especially love. When working your way toward forgiveness, it will help to remember that forgiveness takes courage, and courage comes from love.

Many of my patients have been faced with extremely difficult choices in order to heal emotionally and physically and go on to live fuller lives. They have gotten divorced, ended long-term relationships with friends or family members, or revealed secrets that came with serious consequences. Making major changes like these requires us to move forward in faith, not knowing exactly what the outcome will be but trusting it will work out for the highest good of all concerned. We can't do this if a lack of forgiveness is holding us back and keeping us stuck in the past.

My patient Anna was feeling completely stuck when she first came to see me. She was suffering from persistent insomnia that had gotten so bad, I could see that sleeplessness was at least part of her problem the moment she walked in the room. She was pale, with dark hollows around her eyes, and appeared to be practically dragging herself across the floor. Lack of sleep was especially difficult for her, she explained, because as a young single woman and former model who worked in the fashion industry, appearance was a crucial factor in how she defined herself, how she made her living, and the social environment she was part of every day. Her confidence, self-esteem, psychological wellbeing, social wellbeing, and even her standing at work were on the line. Every time she looked in the mirror and saw the effects of yet another sleepless night written all over her face, she felt at her wits' end.

Despite a measure of understandable fogginess given how long it had been since she had enjoyed a full night's rest, Anna came across as a competent and ambitious young woman. When we began discussing her work, I received my first clue to what might be contributing to her sleep problems. "I like my job," she said, "but it's not the ideal environment for me. The people I work with on a day-to-day basis are all women, and I really prefer working with men."

The statement caught my attention. The notion that she could work better with men than with women struck me as the kind of story someone tells when they are emotionally posturing, which is one of the mechanisms of repression, or pretending a situation isn't causing them to have negative feelings. After all, all women aren't the same, nor are all men, so I suspected there was something about the particular group of women she worked with that bothered her. This suspicion made me want to know more about Anna's workplace, so I began asking her open-ended questions (our way of following the signs—step five). *What specifically do you find difficult about your environment? How do you imagine it would be better if you worked with different people?*

What emerged was a picture of a woman whose work was her life, a situation that would have made her content if only she felt better about her work relationships. Anna lived alone and had no romantic partner. She typically worked from 7:00 a.m. to 7:00 p.m., and her time away from the office consisted mostly of eating, trying to get some sleep, and getting ready to go back to work. Her workplace relationships were her primary ones. Many people don't realize that social relationships, whether among colleagues at work or friends in our personal lives, can be a tremendous source of stress.

Anna was particularly susceptible to this kind of stress because work occupied such a large part of her life. As she described a workplace culture of backstabbing and undermining, it became clear that these primary relationships in her life weren't supportive. What's more, she felt like the "odd girl out" among her peers and was suffering because of it.

The odd girl out often feels self-hatred and doubt. When any group singles out someone through negative attention or ostracizing, it can take a heavy toll on that person's self-esteem. Chronic stress of this nature always has an impact on physical health. As we discussed her situation further, Anna realized she had started feeling targeted at work around the same time she began having trouble sleeping.

The next open-ended question I asked was *If your work, which is such a big part of your life, is the source of so much stress for you, why have you stayed so long?*

The answers tumbled out of her. She blamed the women in her office and admitted she believed that if she left the company, she would be letting them "win." She blamed herself, feeling she ought to be able to manage the situation better and prevail over their pettiness. A polarity had been created, her versus them. She was the good girl and they were the bad girls. The presence of these two opposing sides was creating resistance. The resistant energy had taken up residence in her body and was keeping her stuck in a job that didn't serve her. It was also keeping her body from getting adequate rest.

If Anna wanted to sleep again, she needed to make some changes, and change takes courage. She needed to confront the truth of her situation (by admitting to and embracing her suffering—step seven) so she could change the context of what was happening to her (by assigning new meaning—step eight), thereby shifting from blame to love.

Rather than focusing on whose fault it was, hers or theirs, Anna refocused her energy on loving herself. Once she was able to do this, she realized she deserved to work in a place where she felt supported and could thrive. It took a lot of courage, but she worked on forgiving herself for staying in a corrosive situation for so long.

Once she could forgive herself, Anna went on to work on forgiving her colleagues for the way they had treated her, eventually thanking them in her own thoughts for showing her she wasn't placing enough value on herself and her happiness. But although she forgave them, she didn't let them continue to get away with their behavior. She made the decision to move on, quitting her job. As soon as she did, she was able to sleep well again almost immediately. At the time she quit, she wasn't exactly sure what she would do next, but she gave herself some time to explore her options. For her next job, she used what she had learned at her previous position to be much more thorough in examining the social environment before determining if the job was the right fit for her. She also placed much greater value on establishing positive relationships with the people around her. Eventually she went on to start her own business, where she had even more influence on not just the work she did but the environment in which she worked.

Clarity isn't a single moment of inspiration but a long and winding path that requires many acts of courage along the way—to see things in new ways, to let go when something isn't serving us, to create change even when we aren't sure how things will turn out. Anna did all these, and it took her to a place where her life is much fuller, much freer, and much more fulfilling as a result.

This is what you'll strive for as you try the following forgiveness exercises. You may feel a release the first time or you may need to do them multiple times. Neither outcome is better than the other. There's no pressure or time limit. The only rule is to be persistent. Like clarity itself, forgiveness is a process, so have the courage to stick with it.

"Holding on to anger is like grasping a hot coal with the intent of throwing it at someone else; you are the one who gets burned."

—Buddha

EXERCISE:
The ~~Confession~~ Revelation Booth—Part Two

The confession booth in the Catholic religion is a place where transformation and absolution occur. Those seeking to confess walk into the booth with their sins weighing on their minds and walk out having been granted forgiveness. That's much like what will happen here. In part one of this exercise, which you completed in the last step, you confessed your judgments and transformed them into loving meaning. Now is the time for forgiveness and absolution.

DIRECTIONS

1. Look back at the two columns you created in part one of the ~~Confession~~ Revelation Booth exercise—your judgments and your loving meaning around a specific event in your life that has caused you suffering. Notice how, from left to right, you transformed your challenge into possibilities for learning, growing, and expanding your world.

2. With this transformation in mind, complete the "forgiveness release" that follows:

Dear _____,

I understand that you came into my life as my partner in learning a powerful lesson. You helped me discover my false belief that _____. Even though _____ had to happen for me to understand this, I'm grateful for the gifts it has brought me and how it has uplifted my life in ways such as _____. I understand that this was the best way for me to make this change and that, on the soul level, you chose to help me. I am grateful to you for this gift and know that your actions came from your understanding given the givens at the time. I forgive you and hold my experience in the light of compassion and love. Thank you for being my partner in this healing experience. I release it now and we are both free.

Example: Once again, let's use Gina and her experience with bullying to imagine how someone in a particular set of circumstances might complete this release:

Dear _boy with the video camera,_

I understand that you came into my life as my partner in learning a powerful lesson. You helped me discover my false belief that _I'm not worthy of love or respect._ Even though _a challenging period_ had to happen for me to understand this, I'm grateful for the gifts it has brought me and how it has uplifted my life in ways such as: _I am a much more compassionate and empathetic person, which has helped me deepen my relationships with my husband and daughter. As a physical therapist, it has also helped me to better understand my clients and the pain they are experiencing so that I'm better able to help them, which I believe is my life's purpose._ I understand that this was the best way for me to make this change and that, on the soul level, you chose to help me. I am grateful to you for this gift and know that your actions came from your understanding given the givens at the time. I forgive you and hold my experience in the light of compassion and love. Thank you for being my partner in this healing experience. I release it now and we are both free.

3. This final step is designed to elevate your feeling of release. Get a helium-filled balloon of your choice. You can find them at most dollar stores, party supply stores, or florist shops. Go to a quiet, private place that's special to you. It could be your patio, apartment balcony, backyard, or a remote corner of a park. Read your forgiveness release statement out loud with reverence, respect, and gratitude. When you're finished, release the balloon. Open your arms as wide as they will go. This will encourage a strong sense of expansion. Watch the balloon drift away and feel your burden become lighter as it gets higher and higher and eventually disappears.

EXERCISE:
The Practice of Compassionate Self-Forgiveness*

As I mentioned earlier, the mistake we often make is to focus our forgiveness entirely on the other person, when forgiveness is really about ourselves. Still, there's a difference when the act we're forgiving has been committed by someone else versus an act we have committed against ourselves. The latter tends to be fraught with stronger emotion.

The following template can help you in either situation—forgiving someone else or forgiving yourself—because our relationships with others mirror our relationship with ourselves. When we hold a judgment against someone else, we hold that same judgment against ourselves. In other words, when people do things from time to time that appear to us as insensitive or unkind, it can be read as a clue that we are perhaps acting in an insensitive or unkind way toward ourselves. Otherwise, why would we react so significantly to someone else's careless action? We can blame or rage against the other person, or we can use the situation to serve our own growth and healing. When we choose to thank such a person for the lesson they're teaching us and respond to them with love, we're also making a positive choice to move forward in love rather than bitterness. When we make the loving choice, it's a signal to ourselves that we are worthy of our own kindness, consideration, and loving attention.

Because our relationships with others reflect our relationship with ourselves, when we practice compassionate forgiveness, it's really toward

---

*Used by permission of Drs. Ron and Mary Hulnick and the University of Santa Monica (USM). Drs. Ron and Mary Hulnick are pioneers and innovators in the field of spiritual psychology. As USM's founding faculty and co-directors, they designed the university's extraordinary curriculum in spiritual psychology and they continue to serve as senior faculty for USM.

ourselves that it needs to be directed. This is true even if we are forgiving someone else. All we need in order to engage in this exercise is
ourselves, no matter who the object of forgiveness is. The other person
doesn't need to be in the room with us for it to work. The following template can be used anytime you need to release blame or judgment you're
holding against anyone at all—yourself, or someone else.

DIRECTIONS

1. Think of a child you love. Allow your heart to open. From this
   place, experience the feeling of loving.
   or
   Think of the person you love the most. Allow your heart to
   open, connecting you with your love.
   or
   Place your right hand over your heart as a way of connecting
   with your love.
2. From this heart space, begin moving into compassionate self-
   forgiveness by centering yourself within your self. You may
   want to call on your authentic self as you did on page 60.
3. In the template that follows, simply fill in the blanks of the relevant statements with the name of the person you're thinking
   about, or focus on the alternative version that will help facilitate forgiveness of your own trespasses against yourself.

I forgive myself for judging [person's name or myself] as insensitive, inconsiderate, and unkind.

I forgive myself for judging myself as somehow needing
[person's name]'s approval and acceptance.

I forgive myself for judging myself by taking [person's
name]'s behavior personally.

I forgive myself for judging myself as unworthy of consideration, kindness, and loving attention from myself and others.

I forgive myself for judging myself as unworthy of higher consciousness and greater awareness.

I forgive myself for judging myself as unworthy of God's love or believing I needed to do something to earn it.

4. When you're finished, read the words aloud to yourself. Say them over and over again until you feel your negative emotions recede. You can then return to these words, like a mantra or prayer, anytime the same feelings arise.
5. End by acknowledging the courageous act you have just completed and thanking yourself for your forgiveness.

....

PURPOSE OF COMPASSIONATE SELF-FORGIVENESS

....

1. To heal through the compassionate application of loving to emotional pain
2. To balance inner disturbance through letting go of judgment and surrendering to the love that's our true nature
3. To assist in establishing compassionate self-forgiveness as a positive habit to be exercised as we become aware of our judgments
4. To affirm our awareness that we are worthy and that our true nature is love. Self-forgiveness is compassion in action!

....

Bring Balance to Forgiveness

An important factor in constructing a septic system is the rule that the size of the leach field is directly proportional to the volume of wastewater that runs into it, but inversely proportional to the porosity of the gravel-soil mixture that it's made up of. Basically, this means that a big family will produce a large amount of wastewater, so the leach field needs to be equally large to handle the filtering of so many gallons. However, the gravel-soil mixture of the leach field needs to be denser and less porous, forcing the water to take longer to pass through more levels of filtration before exiting the system.

When we forgive, we allow our negative emotions to pass through the final cleansing stage of the emotional waste management process. They pass through our internal leach field in order to complete the cycle. Emotionally speaking, the porosity of our leach field needs to reflect the size of the trespass we are forgiving. If it's too loose and porous, our emotions pass right through without adequate processing and remain toxic. A good example is when we rush to forgiveness because we feel anger isn't spiritual or because we don't want to hold a grudge against someone we care deeply about, like a child, partner, or parent. Anger can be healthy, a kind of filter of fire through which certain experiences can be cleansed. The things we forgive too quickly often don't stay forgiven. As a result, toxic resentment will fester because we didn't fully process the emotions that were created by the experience that triggered our anger.

On the other hand, if our internal leach field is dense, stoic, and unforgiving, then our emotional filtration system won't have enough porous openings through which emotional waste can be neutralized. The lack of porosity causes buildup, backup, and eventually pollutes our property—or in this case our body, making us sick with disease.

When we jump to forgiveness, or when we are begrudging about it, it's because we're uncomfortable with the negative feelings we have to hold in order to make forgiveness possible. So we resort to those old mechanisms of repression. We emotionally posture, pretending something isn't as difficult as it seems, and forgive quickly but not fully. Or we emotionally armor or shut down, which stops forgiveness in its tracks. We need to take the time to find the middle ground between rushing to forgiveness and rushing past it. As you use the exercises in this step to work toward forgiveness, give yourself the gift of the dignity of your emotional process and let it take as long as it requires.

Restore Your Life Force

We've come a long way together since the start of this book. You've learned what clarity is and how it can help you heal, both psycho-spiritually and physically, so that you can go on to live a healthier, happier, and more fulfilling life. You've come to understand how you have unintentionally been keeping yourself from clarity by let-ting your consciousness become cluttered and clogged with unpro-cessed thoughts and emotions, particularly negative ones that stem from difficult experiences. You've started to confront some of those thoughts and emotions and learned to sit with your doubts and fears so that you can begin to process them. You've come to embrace suf-fering for all the possibilities of change and expansion it can bring. You've learned to create new, more empowering, more truthful meanings for the things in your life you struggle with and that cause you suffering. And you've practiced forgiveness for your own sake, so that you don't have to remain cluttered and clogged any longer. All this has been part of the process of creating clarity.

You've done a lot of work on yourself thus far, breaking down old habits and beliefs and clearing space in your consciousness. The step where you embraced suffering marked the end of the catabolic or breaking-down phase in your emotional cycle. It was a turning point, like the winter solstice. We are now in the anabolic phase when your days will begin growing longer and be filled with an increasing amount of light.

In this step, you'll spend some time preparing yourself for a brand-new spring. You'll do this by looking at different ways to restore your energy and put yourself in a healing frame of mind so you can get the most out of this anabolic phase in your emotional cycle and build yourself back up again. By creating an emotional waste management system for yourself and using it to clear out the psycho-spiritual muck that has been holding you back, you have created space inside yourself where new things—new ways of thinking, new ways of being, new opportunities that can enhance and expand your life—can take root and grow. That's why, at the end of this step, you will focus on picturing the wonderful possibilities of what might come rushing into the empty space you've created. Time for a bit of inspiration!

Feel Better to Get Better

We don't live in a physical body disconnected from what we think and feel. We exist in a mind + body system where both parts work synergistically. Therefore the best approach as we work toward restoring ourselves is to treat both mind and body together.

To give an example of how intimately the mind and body are connected, we need only to think of what it feels like when we're frightened by something and our fight-or-flight response kicks in. When this happens, we feel our heart rate rise, our breath quicken, our bodies start to perspire, and perhaps experience a heightening of our senses so that we become hyperaware of our surroundings. Inside our bodies, the stress hormone cortisol rises rapidly, while much of the blood that feeds our organs is diverted to our arms and legs, preparing us to run to safety or fight for our lives. Resources are diverted from bodily functions that aren't absolutely necessary in an emergency, such as our digestion and immune function. When running for your life, digesting your breakfast can wait. In moments of fear, these biological changes happen instantaneously, and they're all triggered by our thoughts and the feelings these thoughts generate.

Stress of any kind sets off the same survival reaction in the body. This is also the case when the stress isn't caused by a life-or-death situation. Our bodies don't register a distinction between feeling stressed because we're fleeing a burning building or feeling stressed because we're overwhelmed at work. The biological changes that happen as a result are basically the same. Because immune suppression is one of those biological changes, chronic stress leads to a breakdown of the body and makes us vulnerable to diseases of all kinds.

The late Dr. Candace Pert of the National Institute of Mental Health discovered that every time we think a thought, a molecule is created in our bodies. Whether those chemical molecules benefit or harm our health depends on how those thoughts make us feel. Informally, she called these the "molecules of emotion," and wrote a groundbreaking book by the same name, because the feelings we experience change our body chemistry from moment to moment. Each of our cells has thousands of receptors on its surface. When emotionally generated molecules come in contact with our cells, they find the receptors that match their chemical composition and attach to them, then enter the cell with specific instructions on how it should perform. If those chemical instructions were generated from feelings of love, joy, and relaxation, then the cells will respond by working toward optimal function and balance. If, however, the chemical message is one of fear, frustration, resentment, or another stress-generating emotion, the cells will respond accordingly, moving into protection mode by suppressing healthy functions and possibly enhancing disease-related functions based on the instructions they've been given. Because our feelings are so complex, we can cause an infinite number of changes in our bodies by changing the way we think and react to our emotions.

This understanding of the mind-body system helps explain why clarity is so crucial. If we want to heal—psycho-spiritually from past trauma or current difficulties, or physically from discomfort or disease—we need to learn how we can make ourselves feel better. We can heal from the inside out because our bodies contain an incredible pharmacy that can produce countless healing chemical combinations modern science can't even conceive of. When coupled with necessary lifestyle changes, these internal healing compounds can be as effective as drugs or surgery, and in most cases more so. The act of thinking is to practice brain chemistry and, by association, body chemistry.

When we hear about cases of spontaneous healing in the medical profession, the patients have nearly always used their minds to get well. Some think of spontaneous healing as hocus-pocus or wishful thinking, but documented cases arise again and again. A search through the medical literature the world over will eventually reveal that someone, somewhere has recovered from every so-called incurable illness known to humans. Dig a little deeper and it becomes clear the recovery depended on the motivation of the patient and their understanding of the primary role they play in their own healing process.

When American diplomat Norman Cousins was diagnosed with ankylosing spondylitis, a painful and crippling disease that disintegrates the connective tissue in the spine and the rest of the body, he did two things. He made some significant lifestyle changes, and he chose to use his mind and emotions to start generating some very powerful healing compounds inside his own body. His excruciating pain made it virtually impossible to sleep, but he discovered almost by accident that if he watched something on TV that was funny enough to make him laugh out loud before he went to bed, he could get through the night relatively well. This was the 1960s, and he happened to know the producers of the comedy-reality show *Candid Camera*, which he loved very much and really got him laughing. Fortunately he was able to get reels of the show and watched several episodes daily, using laughter as a powerful tool for recovery from this otherwise incurable disease. Cousins would later document his dramatic recovery in his book *Anatomy of an Illness*.

Renowned cancer surgeon and author of *Love, Medicine & Miracles*, Dr. Bernie Siegel, shared yet another inspiring example in his book when he told the story of his patient Arthur who, after being diagnosed with advanced-stage cancer, was given less than a year to live and sent home to get his affairs in order. Five years later Dr. Siegel ran into Arthur in the grocery store and was astonished to see him looking very much alive and well. When Dr. Siegel asked his patient what had happened, Arthur reminded him of the advice the doctor had given him after he'd revealed his diagnosis. Because he believed his patient had only a short time left, Dr. Siegel had told Arthur to make it the best six to twelve months of his life. Arthur had taken the advice literally. He went home and quit the job he'd never really liked, booked himself on a cruise he'd always wanted to take, and began piano lessons, which was something else he'd always wanted to do. After six months of this new life, Arthur said he was feeling so good that he decided he didn't have to die. Five years later, he was in great health and hadn't been sick once during the interim.

Flabbergasted, Dr. Siegel had his staff follow up with the families of many patients he'd long assumed had passed away only to discover that nearly 20 percent of them were still alive years later and completely healthy. "There are no incurable diseases, only incurable people," Dr. Siegel concluded in *Love, Medicine & Miracles*.

Recovering from an extraordinary illness or extraordinary life circumstances requires an exceptional patient who is willing to make the kinds of life changes and do the necessary mental work integral to healing. No pharmacy, surgeon, therapist, or guru can do that work for you. So let's start looking at what more you can do to feel and to be extraordinary.

....

FEEL BETTER BY TAKING A SOOTHING BATH

....

Sometimes simple things can make all the difference. I often suggest to patients that they take baths to reduce stress and help them relax and rejuvenate. The following prescription will enhance the experience:

- Add five drops of lavender essential oil to a teaspoon of natural bath gel and add to a warm bath.
- Add a cup of Epsom salts if you like. The minerals in the salts can help detoxify the body.

....

Selfless Selfishness and Spiritual Nutrition

The silence and peaceful solitude inside a mother's womb facilitate the nourishment and growth of the fetus. Long after we're born and for the rest of our lives, we continue to need healing, nourishment, and growth not only for our bodies but for our minds as well. Even so, most of us do little or nothing to re-create a womb-like environment for ourselves, a place where we can go to relax, recharge, nourish our soul, and heal from the emotional pollution of our lives. When we neglect ourselves in this primal way, the soul is starved, and when we are malnourished spiritually we become ill physically.

Selfless people, more often women, have an especially difficult time with self-nourishment. By selfless, I mean people who are constantly putting themselves last on the to-do list—or worse, not putting themselves on it at all. They cancel their own plans in order to help a friend move house, work an extra shift so someone can take the day off, organize the church bake sale, run the PTA fundraiser, chauffeur the kids to basketball and ballet practice, and do about ten other things simply because no one else will. Individual acts of kindness are always appreciated, but obsessively helping others in a way that results in neglecting our own needs leaves us emotionally depleted and physically weakened. Over time it is a prescription for unhappiness and illness.

Creating a womb—a time and place or environment that's just for us—is an essential way to nourish our souls, process emotions, and experience spiritual growth. How and where aren't nearly as important as making a point to do it on a regular basis. I recommend at least once or twice each week for 10 to 20 minutes at a time.

Creating a womb space could be as simple as finding a chair you love in your home and making that the place where you go to read a book, listen to music, meditate, or anything else that restores you. You can pick a spot under your favorite tree in the backyard or a room in your house that you love but rarely have time to enjoy. You might carve out your own cave in the garage, a shed in the backyard, or the basement if that's what works. It doesn't matter where you go or what you do as long as it has emotional resonance for you and you won't be disturbed for at least 10 minutes.

It might seem contrary to the natural impulses of some, but in life it's crucial to serve ourselves first. When we take the time to fill ourselves up with the joy of what matters to us, then we have more than enough love and joy to give to everyone else. Spending time doing things only for ourselves will make us better parents, partners, friends, coworkers, and so on. Feeding the soul is so important that I call it "spiritual nutrition" and actually prescribe it for my patients as an essential tool for good psycho-spiritual and physical wellbeing. I also refer to it as "selfless selfishness" because giving to ourselves first is one of the greatest gifts we could ever give to those we love.

Taking care of ourselves, especially in such a personal way, isn't always easy. Do your best to resist false feelings of guilt and create an environment where you can pursue activities that are especially pleasurable for you, things that put you back in touch with the parts of you that *aren't* a wife, husband, parent, boss, employee, and so on. When we learn the art of self-love in this way, even in the smallest, briefest moments, we incubate our souls in preparation for the birth of a greater, truer version of ourselves that we always knew we could be.

EXERCISE:
My-Time Meditation

The following meditation is written in the first person and is meant to reinforce the value of carving out a regular time and space that's just for you. It's meant to reinforce the message that, while it may feel selfish to do so, you will be practicing a kind of selfless selfishness that will only enhance your capacity for giving to others.

Ideally, read the following words aloud. I find that when people read things aloud using the first person narrative, they don't merely listen to the words, they take ownership of the concepts. It helps make it more real and encourages them to apply the information directly to themselves. At the same time, by using the first person and saying it aloud, there's an automatic feeling of commitment that comes into play. People are more inspired and motivated to move into action.

Find a quiet place and read the following words aloud to yourself. Repeat them if you feel inspired to do so:

I love myself, therefore I make my own needs and happiness a priority in my life. I commit to taking time to do things I love away from my present obligations to fill myself back up with loving positive energy after giving so much to others. Filling myself up with love in this way is healing and prevents me from becoming depleted emotionally and energetically, which can lead to disease and illness. Regardless of how busy my schedule may be, I know it's essential that I schedule several 15-to-30-minute sessions of personal time for myself throughout the week to engage in something I enjoy or that holds meaning for me in a personal way. I also create a space in my home where I can go to relax and partake in activities that bring joy to my heart and peace to my soul. In this way it's easier to keep myself on my to-do list and feed my soul with positive healing energy on a regular basis.

I don't define myself by what I can give to others. I too deserve my own love. When I fill myself up to overflowing with things that bring joy to me, I have more love to give others in my life. When I'm rejuvenated with self-love like this, I become more powerful, passionate, and attentive in every role I fill. Giving love to myself and filling my heart up first isn't selfish, but the most selfless gift I could ever give to those who are dear to me. They love me and want me to do this for myself.

When I regularly take time to address my own needs and desires, I flood my body with the healing energy of the love I feel for what I'm doing and either speed recovery or reinforce my existing health. The more I take time to love myself by doing things I love to do, the more I'm revealing my authentic self and living as the person I was always meant to be.

The Healing Power of Nature

Part of any healing, restorative regime must include regular connections with the earth. This was one of the things my wife Sherry and I had in mind when we moved our practice from the city to the countryside outside of Los Angeles, with its rolling hills, long vistas, and relative quiet. The healing energy in this kind of environment is powerful. To enhance this energy, we created a Zen garden leading up to the front door so patients could spend time in nature as they waited for their appointments. Long after their appointments are over, we find them relaxing and socializing in the garden.

Many people gravitate toward nature instinctively, but there's also scientific evidence supporting the idea that nature has healing properties. German scientist Wolfgang Ludwig was one of the first to study the earth-mind connection as part of his research on the components of a healthy environment. Through this work, he discovered that the earth's frequency, known as the Schumann resonance after the professor who first discovered it, can be easily measured in the countryside or at the beach, whereas it's impossible to measure in the city where our civilization's electromagnetic signals interfere with or obscure it.

In 1963 Dr. Rutger Wever of the Max Planck Institute in Germany built on Ludwig's findings when he recruited several students to live in an underground bunker that screened out the earth's frequency. During their four weeks there, the students reported experiencing heightened levels of stress, emotional upset, and migraine headaches. However, after leaving the bunker and being exposed to the earth's frequency once again, they recovered rapidly from all their symptoms.

Thanks in part to scientific research showing its benefits, contact with nature is also used in many therapeutic settings. Environmental psychologist Roger Ulrich and a team of researchers reviewed the medical records of patients recovering from surgery at a hospital in Pennsylvania and found that those who could see views of trees and greenery from their beds healed a full day faster on average than patients with views of brick walls. In addition, those patients with nature views needed significantly less pain medication and had fewer post-surgical complications. The results were so striking that many hospitals began to consider gardens a crucial part of their design, making them part of their offering to both patients and employees. Further research from a team at the University of Essex in the United Kingdom, which studied the effects of nature on people suffering depression, found that 90 percent of subjects felt a higher level of self-esteem and nearly 75 percent felt less depressed after a simple walk in a country park.

These are just a few examples of a wealth of evidence linking nature with benefits to our health and wellbeing. Taken together, the research makes it clear that it's essential to maintain a consistent connection with the natural world as a way to nourish both our bodies and souls.

EXERCISE:
Plug Into the Natural World

When you need to restore and recharge, think about the natural world as a place where you can literally plug yourself in. This can mean getting out into the actual countryside or spending time at a local park or beach, depending on where you live and what works best for you. Wherever you go to connect with nature, keep the following points in mind to get the most out of the experience:

1. Be sure to spend at least some of your nature time walking barefoot and lying in the grass or sand. Make as much bodily contact with the earth as possible. Sleeping on the ground, as you might do when camping, is also highly rejuvenating. Some sports teams have been known to have their players sleep on the ground the night before a big event to recharge their energy.

2. Remember to steer clear of any devices that might interrupt your connection to the earth's frequency. Cell phones, Wi-Fi, microwave ovens, radio transmissions, TV antennas, baby monitors, and countless other devices emit their own electromagnetic frequencies that short-circuit our connection to the earth's natural vibration.

3. If you can spend some time in nature several times a week and pair it with several gadget detoxes throughout the month, you'll be well on your way to recharging your mind, body, and spirit. (See instructions in the sidebar that follows.)

GADGET UNSATURATION AND REJUVENATION UNINTERRUPTED (GURU)

In our world today it has become quite common to develop an unhealthy attachment to our cell phones or other electronic devices. Recent research shows that cell phone use can be addictive, triggering the release of serotonin and dopamine in the brain, which are the same "feel good" chemicals connected with addictions to smoking, drinking, and gambling. Even if you aren't overly attached to your gadgets, they may still be disrupting your clarity and peace of mind. All electronic devices emit an electromagnetic field, which can affect our bodies and minds in ways we don't yet fully understand. Little research has been done, for example, on how long-term cell phone use affects a person's health. At the same time, the way we use these devices changes the way we think and exercise our minds, and not always for the better. For all these reasons, I highly recommend planning regular time in your schedule to take a break from your gadgets. Try the following tips and see what sort of effect GURU has on you.

1. Go to the nearest electronics store and get a battery-operated alarm clock. Then, instead of using your cell phone as an alarm, leave it in another room overnight for ten days. Studies have shown that people exposed to radiation from cell phones take longer to fall asleep, so you may just find yourself more rested in the mornings. What's more, you will have taken a first step toward becoming less reliant on your device.

2. Now that you have removed one attachment to your cell phone, let's try another. Identify the top five people you call most often and memorize their phone numbers before deleting them from your phone. As modern society has become more and more reliant on technology, many of us have stopped exercising our memories on a regular basis. This is a problem because research suggests that when we don't use it, we lose it, and lack of use may even contribute to dementia and Alzheimer's later in life.

3. Once you have begun to exercise your memory, take it to the next level. Next time you go grocery shopping, instead of keeping your list on your phone, memorize it. Research has shown that people are less likely to overspend when they memorize their shopping lists rather than write them down. It seems that when you use your memory in this way, you also turn on the analytical part of your brain and are able to make better decisions in the moment.

4. Spend a few days paying attention to how you use your phone and other devices and create your own opportunities to break your reliance on them. As you do this, remember the KISS principle, which stands for Keep It Simply Simple. This means looking for opportunities that can be easily executed and worked into your regular routine, like finding your own way to locations you have been to before

rather than relying on GPS, or memorizing your appointment calendar for the day. Simple tricks like these can have a profound psycho-spiritual effect over time and help you gain greater clarity.

....

Imagining the Future You Want

Through my studies in microbiology and electrochemistry, I became familiar with the work of Dmitri Mendeleev. This Russian chemist is known to everyone who studies these disciplines because in the 1860s he created something used to this day—the periodic table of elements. This chart organized all the physical building blocks of our universe into a cohesive, logical order by atomic weight. The table included elements like gold, silver, lead, argon, neon, helium, and every other mineral, metal, and gas known at the time.

While the table was incredibly useful, it had a problem. Wherever Mendeleev couldn't find a transitional substance that connected two elements, he left a blank space. At the time, there were no known elements with the right atomic weights to fit into those spaces and make the chart whole. While his table worked well for certain kinds of scientific research, detractors were quick to point out these gaps. When questioned about them, Mendeleev was unconcerned. His response was, "Indeed the holes exist, but that doesn't mean the elements don't. We just have to look for them."

Today every one of those elements has been discovered and the table is complete. Mendeleev gives us a perfect example of how the power of imagination can bring things into being. Just because we can't prove that what we desire exists doesn't mean it isn't there. We just haven't found it yet. Or perhaps it hasn't found us.

Mendeleev's way of creating the periodic table has always inspired me. His powerful leap of faith and use of imagination to manifest what no one else could conceive of are things I try to impress on my patients. "As people think in their hearts, so they are in life," as it says in the Bible (Proverb 23:7, paraphrased). Mendeleev didn't worry about how certain elements would take shape as he painted his picture. Instead he trusted the process, and eventually the "how" revealed itself. This unfettered way of thinking is something that can inspire you as you look toward the future and work to create a life you truly want to lead.

EXERCISE:
Create Your Ideal Scene

Mendeleev had his chart, holes and all. You, too, can create a map of where you want to go. It doesn't matter if there are holes or if you don't know how this or that could possibly happen. Just paint a picture in your mind of what you want in as much detail as possible.

Once you've pictured your ideal scene, write it down, say it aloud to yourself, or even record yourself describing it so you can play it back later. Choose whichever method feels most natural to you, but remember to be specific. For example, don't simply say, "I want to feel better." What does feeling better look like to you? You might say, "I am feeling joy and full of love as I easily walk, with strength and vitality, on the white-sand beaches of Tahiti with my beloved husband." This gives the universe something to work with!

Do your best to finish your ideal scene with a thought such as, "Like this or something better, for the highest good of all concerned." While it's important to picture your scene in as much detail as possible, it's equally important not to think of all those details as requirements so that the universe can bring you what it's been working on for you. Would you argue if the universe created your ideal scene but it happened to be on the white, sandy beaches of the Bahamas rather than Tahiti? No, me neither.

Plan Time to Restore

Keep in mind that there are countless ways to restore. Some people meditate or practice yoga. Others listen to music, and in fact numerous studies link music and health. To give just one example, see some of the amazing results of research into the effects of Mozart's work in the following sidebar. I've also included in the appendix a number of ways to restore and open your spirit. "The 'Being' List" includes books to read and movies to watch, and "Meditation Moments" provides quick inspirations that take no more than a minute to do.

....

THE MOZART EFFECT
....

While nearly all music has an effect on the mind and body, Mozart's compositions seem to carry an impact that sets them apart from others. Because of their ability to heighten creativity and foster healing for many listeners, the phenomenon has even been dubbed the Mozart Effect. The following are some of the amazing results that have come to light from studying this curious phenomenon:

- A study published in the *Journal of Cardiothoracic Surgery* showed that music by Mozart reduced the rejection of heart transplants in mice and extended the functioning time before the transplant failed.
- A study published in *Pediatrics* showed that playing Mozart to premature infants in the neonatal intensive

care unit (NICU) supported weight gain and accelerated growth.

- Research conducted at the Center for the Neurobiology of Learning and Memory in Irvine, California, showed that after listening to 10 minutes of Mozart's Sonata for Two Pianos in D Major, students increased their spatial IQ scores by eight points or more for up to 15 minutes after hearing the music.

The method isn't as important as your conscious intention. Remember to set aside regular time to restore yourself. It's important to make this a part of your regular habits, but it's particularly important when you're focusing on the kind of work you've been pursuing in this book. Always remember that a life of clarity is a life of balance.

Mind + Body, The Complete Clarity Cleanse

Two of the earliest steps along this path to clarity were about cleansing the body through five days of the Intentional Unsaturation Diet and cleansing the mind through the PEW 12 exercise. Now that we're nearing the end of our journey together, we are going to put these two together in a more advanced version, the Complete Clarity Cleanse.

In the previous steps, you cleansed first one and then the other. Now you are going to cleanse both at the same time. It's important to do both because many people, whether consciously or not, still follow the theory of "mind-body dualism" put forth by the French philosopher René Descartes in the 17th century. Building on ideas from ancient Greece, he argued in his now famous dualist thesis that the nature of the mind is separate and distinct from the nature of the body. As he wrote in his *Sixth Meditation*, "On the one hand I have a clear and distinct idea of myself, in so far as I am simply a thinking, non-extended thing, and on the other hand I have a distinct idea of body, in so far as this is simply an extended, non-thinking thing. And accordingly, it is certain that I am really distinct from my body, and can exist without it."

The concept of mind-body dualism was conceived of centuries ago and was based on a very limited understanding of human anatomy and the human mind. DNA, for example, which contains the genetic code of all living organisms, wasn't identified by scientists until the latter half of the 19th century, and its double helix structure wasn't understood until the 1950s. The word *psychiatry*, referring to the study of the human mind, wasn't coined until 1808, more than 100 years after Descartes' death. His dualist ideas have nonetheless persisted for generations, and today it's still common for people to see themselves as two separate, even conflicting parts— body versus mind.

As I hope I've made clear by this point in our journey together, I don't believe in this separation, nor do many who study the nature of the mind and body today. In the last step, I mentioned a number of the many documented cases of so-called spontaneous healing, where patients used their minds to help them recover from critical illnesses. These stories are just the tip of the iceberg.

In the 20th and 21st centuries, there has been ample research to document the mind-body connection. The most widely known example came from American cardiologists Meyer Friedman and R. H. Rosenman in the 1950s. The two doctors were puzzled about why their waiting room chairs were wearing out so quickly, particularly on the edges of the seats and arms. They consulted an upholsterer who determined that their patients were quite literally sitting on the edge of their seats, clutching their armrests as they waited for their names to be called and their fates to be revealed. Friedman and Rosenman wondered whether their patients could really be so mentally anxious that they couldn't contain their anxiety physically. Following subsequent research, they discovered that anxious and restless personality traits were common among people with heart disease. As a result they coined the term "type A personality."

More recently the Morsani College of Medicine at the University of South Florida has produced similar research into Parkinson's disease, which found that the majority of patients in the study displayed the same personality traits of being overly cautious and fearful of taking risks. Research from Duke University Medical Center has shown that in addition to anxiousness, depression, hostility, and anger also play a significant role in developing heart disease. In fact the more these personality traits are present, the higher the risk factor for acquiring the disease.

An important purpose of this cleanse is to help you start seeing yourself as a whole being—body + mind making up two parts of one whole—so that you can better understand yourself. The more familiar you are with this process, the more it will become second nature to notice how your emotions affect you physically and to examine your physical symptoms or illnesses for their mental or emotional roots. As you place your focus on healing emotionally, physical healing will follow as a byproduct. This is the approach that saved my life years ago when I was facing cancer. Through self-knowledge and clarity, it can save yours as well.

Preparing for the Complete Clarity Cleanse

Instead of seeing the body and mind as separate or opposing forces, I like to think of the body as the theater of the mind. It's where our inner drama, which takes place within our minds, shows up in the outside world, as well as where unresolved issues show up in the body as disease. The steps that you've nearly made your way through are nothing more than a means of becoming masterful at processing, expelling, and recovering from that inner drama so that it doesn't fester and manifest in your body.

As an antidote to a Cartesian way of thinking, we're now going to bring together the two parts of the Clarity Cleanse into a single ten-day cleanse—the Intentional Unsaturation Diet (step two), and the Purge Emotional Writing exercise for cleansing the mind of negative energy (step three). This will help you process and expel any issues that have come up since you began this process, while also helping to reinforce a de-differentiation and integration of mind and body. The earlier versions were merely introductions to these cleansing rituals to get you started. The Complete Clarity Cleanse will go deeper and require your full focus and participation, so plan to start it when you have time in your schedule to really dedicate to the process. With this in mind, you'll also want to plan to set aside extra time in the morning or whenever is most convenient for you to complete the various exercises. (See the checklist at the end of this step for a more complete schedule.)

When it comes to your meal planning for the ten-day Intentional Unsaturation Diet, you can once again consult the appendix for the tables and recipes from the goop test kitchen for help. You will have to wean yourself off caffeine before starting, as you did in step two, so begin that process a few days to a few weeks before your target start date for the cleanse, depending on how much caffeine you are used to drinking. The Complete Clarity Cleanse asks that you fast for a full day on day six of the IU Diet. When considering a start date for this version of the cleanse, you may want to look ahead to day six to ensure that it's a light day, preferably even a day you have off work or when your childcare duties are less than usual, so that you don't find yourself getting overly tired. (You'll find more information about fasting in the coming pages.)

Most importantly, get yourself prepared for the Complete Clarity Cleanse by setting a clear, *positive* intention that accurately describes what you would like to get out of the experience. (Refer back to the intention-setting exercise in step one to help you set a new intention.) As you set your intention, it's helpful to remember that cleansing brings negative energy to the surface in the form of unhappy thoughts or uncomfortable feelings so that you can metabolize it. You want to be ready for this, but it's not where you should focus your attention. A positive intention you might set for your cleanse would be to focus attention on yourself (a selfless selfishness) and your wellbeing, or to facilitate a greater and more balanced connection between your mind and body. By setting a positive intention at the outset, you're much more likely to have a positive experience during the cleanse.

THE COMPLETE CLARITY CLEANSE PREPARATION CHECKLIST

☑ This cleanse will require your full focus and participation for ten consecutive days, so plan to start it when you have time in your schedule to dedicate to the process.

☑ The Complete Clarity Cleanse includes a fast for one full day on day six. If possible, plan to make that day a light one, with few activities and minimal stress.

☑ Prepare for the Intentional Unsaturation Diet by weaning yourself off caffeine if necessary, as you did in step two. Refer to the information on page 70 if you would like suggestions for how to do this.

☑ Plan to set aside extra time, in the mornings or whenever is most convenient for you during the day, to complete your exercises. (See the checklist at the end of this step for more.)

☑ Consult the tables and recipes from the goop test kitchen in the appendix for help with meal planning.

☑ Set a positive intention for what you would like to get out of your ten days on the Complete Clarity Cleanse.

....

Cleanse the Mind: PEW 12 and PEW 12-D

The PEW 12 exercise you learned in step three is a great exercise to return to anytime you're going through a trying time in your life. For the next ten days, you are going to resume the PEW 12 exercise but with one modification. Instead of daily, you are going to write every other day. On the alternate days you will engage in the PEW 12-D exercise that follows, which will ask you to release negative energy in a similar way, but through speaking rather than writing (the D stands for dialogue).

As you practice this new exercise, don't be surprised if your emotions come out in more intense ways than you are used to. I once had a patient I'll call Andrea who came to me because she had been diagnosed with tongue cancer. The treatment her oncologist recommended was to have a large section of her tongue cut out, but the idea horrified her. She had an 11-year-old daughter to think about, and she had only recently started a new romantic relationship following a difficult divorce. She wanted to be able to talk with the people in her life, to eat food, to enjoy these basics of everyday living. Losing her tongue would have changed all that.

As I talked with Andrea about her illness, I discovered she had been diagnosed with tongue cancer on the exact day her divorce had been finalized. This seemed like a cruel joke to her at the time, but to me it was a sign we needed to dig deeper. I asked her to tell me more about the divorce. She described a relationship that was largely happy until she gave birth to her now 11-year-old daughter. She had been thrilled about becoming a mother, but her husband reacted unexpectedly. Suddenly he didn't find his wife attractive anymore.

When Andrea finally got up the nerve to talk with him about how he felt, he responded, "How can I have sex with you now that your vagina is so big?" Something broke in Andrea's heart when she heard this.

After that conversation, the thought of any kind of sexual contact between the two of them, particularly the oral sex her husband now preferred, made Andrea literally gag. She even started biting her tongue as a way of biting back her words and not voicing the hurt she felt so intensely but didn't know how to process. When the relationship eventually dissolved, she was awarded primary custody of their daughter and planned to move on.

I wasn't surprised that Andrea's cancer showed up after she had put some distance between herself and her relationship. It often takes time for our emotions to catch up to us following a trauma. It's a bit like being stabbed. When that kind of bodily trauma happens, we go into fight-or-flight mode as our adrenaline kicks in. As a result we don't fully feel the pain until we calm down and the adrenaline recedes. Andrea didn't feel the full effects of her trauma until her life started to calm down and she was safely away from the draining effect of her marriage.

When I first met Andrea she had a lot of stored-up negativity that was bursting to come out. When she did the PEW 12-D exercise in my office, she became so loud and violent while communicating with her former husband that I had to take her outside to a grassy area behind my office so she wouldn't disturb the patients in nearby rooms. Although her husband wasn't physically present, she was picturing him so clearly and communicating such deep feelings that her emotions quickly rose to a level that caught us both by surprise. Afterward she was completely exhausted, but she understood the power of what she had done. She had released into the ether much of the stored-up negative energy that had been weighing her down for years.

You too may feel tired, even exhausted or spent, after you've finished this exercise, so it's best to set aside enough time (10 to 20 minutes minimum, and up to 90 minutes if needed) not just to complete the exercise but also to recover from the experience afterward rather than running off to your next appointment. Think of it like the post-op period following surgery, where the goal is simply to rest and recover. Before starting the exercise, it's a good idea to gather any items that will help you do this, like a blanket to wrap yourself in, some soothing music, candles, or warm tea.

Instead of feeling tired, you may find yourself feeling lighter and freer following the exercise. The experience will be different for everyone, but know that the effect is cumulative. The more you do it, the more negative energy you will release and the better you will feel in the long run. Following this cleanse, you can continue to do the exercise anytime you feel you need to discharge negative energy, as long as you give yourself enough time to recover afterward.

Andrea eventually felt better and was able to keep most of her tongue. Over the course of our work together, the tumor shrank to the point where her surgeon needed only to cut out a small portion. The surgeon was then able to use some of the muscle in Andrea's non-dominant hand to rebuild that part of the tongue, leaving her able to eat normally and speak her mind whenever she felt like it.

EXERCISE:
Purge Emotional Dialogue (PEW 12-D)

This exercise is similar to Purge Emotional Writing except that the D stands for dialogue. Instead of writing about your emotions, you're going to speak them aloud in a directed way.

DIRECTIONS

1. Begin by finding a chair (or chairs) and imagining the person (or people) associated with your pain sitting in it. Some find it easier to address a photograph of the person while others simply use their imagination.

2. Set a timer for 12 minutes. Then begin telling the person you are picturing how deeply hurt you feel and how you have suffered as a consequence of their behavior. Completely unload your pent-up emotions as if the person were sitting right there in front of you.

3. Let your rising energy guide you and move you around the room. The more you engage your body, the more negative energy you will expel, so don't be afraid to raise your voice, wave your arms, hit a pillow, or perform any other gestures that come naturally to you.

4. Continue in this way until the timer goes off. At the end of the allotted time, it's important to reset your emotional frequency and replenish your positive energy. Do this by listening to some beautiful music, going for a walk in nature, or doing something else that brings you peace. (See step ten if you want more ideas on how to restore.)

Things to Remember

You may use lots of powerful, negatively charged words during this process to dispel pain, but remember to *never direct them toward yourself.* Self-judgment isn't an act of self-love and will only cause you to internalize more of the negative energy this exercise aims to release.

Although forgiveness is an important part of the clarity process, it's a separate step. (You can return to the exercises in step nine following this cleanse if issues come up that call for forgiveness.) This exercise is about purging negative emotions, so don't censor yourself. Remember that you have every right to feel whatever you are feeling. To rid yourself of those feelings is an act of love and self-care. Be kind to yourself by allowing yourself to be in your own truth in every moment of this process.

Prescription

Over the course of ten days, perform this exercise every other day, alternating with PEW 12. The exercise can be done at any time during the day. Just make sure you plan adequate time to recover and restore after you've finished. If you find yourself bringing up a lot of negative energy, you may want to continue performing both PEW 12 exercises beyond the ten-day mark. For many of my patients who could benefit from additional cleansing, I recommend regular PEW 12 exercises, alternating between the two for a full three months.

Cleanse the Body

During the same period you are doing your PEW 12 exercises, you will also be resuming your Intentional Unsaturation Diet, this time for ten days. Engaging in these two rituals simultaneously will allow you to cleanse and lighten mind and body all at once. Because the body and mind are one system, cleansing one supports the cleansing of the other. The foods on the IU Diet not only help clear blockages in our digestive systems to get them moving more smoothly, they also support mental flexibility. (For example, vitamin B, present in high doses in sardines, affects our thinking—see page 67 of step two.)

For the Complete Clarity Cleanse, you will remain on the IU Diet for ten full days, one of which will be a day of fasting. You will work up to that day, gradually reducing your food intake so that you aren't overly hungry or tired.

When we fast, we take part in a holy ritual that has long been a tradition in many world religions, such as Yom Kippur in Judaism, Ramadan in Islam, and Lent for Catholics. As we saw earlier, as we've become more secular as a society we've lost some of these rituals that served as regular reminders to look inward and focus on restoring our bodies and spirits. Fasting and reflection helped people find and maintain balance, which can be so difficult to achieve in modern life, when so many of us suffer from being overstressed, overtired, and oversaturated.

I once had a patient whose work as an actor had him traveling the globe more often than he was at home. As a result he was constantly getting sick—nothing major, just a respiratory infection here, a gastrointestinal illness there. The doctors he consulted would pump him full of medication so he could keep going, keep performing, keep promoting his projects, and keep traveling as his work required. Cumulatively, these bouts of illness and the remedies prescribed for them were taking their toll on his health. When he told me about his problem, the first thing I suggested was that he find a day during the week when he was less busy than usual and make that a day of fasting. He had so much going on that his mind, body, and immune system were overtaxed. He needed something he could do on a regular basis to help him restore balance.

The patient chose Mondays, when he rarely worked, as a day when he would drink only water, eat nothing, and focus on getting some rest. The effect was almost immediate. He felt better, stronger, and less run-down. Over the long term his immune function improved and he has been getting sick much less often. He says that fasting has not only helped improve his health, it's also had a positive impact on his creativity and his overall outlook on life. He was so inspired that he has made fasting a regular part of his weekly schedule.

I'm not asking you to fast weekly for the rest of your life, but I am going to ask you to try a day of fasting on day six of the ten-day IU Diet. Leading up to this, you should plan to stop eating for a full twelve hours between dinner and breakfast the next morning, just like you did in step two. This means that if you typically have breakfast around 7:00 a.m., plan to stop eating after 7:00 p.m. in the evenings. This will create an even balance, a sort of yin to your yang throughout each day, 12 hours on and 12 hours off. This schedule will also help prepare you for your day of fasting where you will only drink water and consume no food. As I mentioned in your preparation checklist, it's best if you plan for your full day of fasting to fall at a time during the week when you are less busy than usual.

Ten-Day Intentional Unsaturation Diet (IU Diet)

Permitted Foods

Meat (for days one to two, nine to ten): all poultry, fish, shellfish, and egg whites
Vegetables: no restrictions
Fruit: all fresh varieties, no dried

Emphasized Foods

Apples: only pink or red, sliced or grated and allowed to brown in open air
Sardines: fresh or canned in olive oil (smoked are okay)
Brown rice: one to two cups daily

Lemon water: start each day with a large glass, per the instructions on page 72

Fermented foods, such as kimchi, sauerkraut, miso, tempeh, kefir, and kombucha

Foods to Avoid

Sweeteners of any kind
All nuts and nut products
Egg yolks
Dairy
Vinegar
Mustard
Legumes (including soybeans and soy products)
Dried fruit
All oils except olive oil
Caffeine
Alcohol

Ten-Day IU Diet Calendar

Days one to two: eat any foods from permitted foods category.

Day three: don't eat any animal protein except sardines, otherwise eat any foods from permitted foods category.

Days four to five: eat only brown rice, apples, and sardines. Eat as many apples and sardines as desired. Apples should be eaten only when they turn brown from being exposed to air. Grate or slice apples to help oxidize them. Apples can be eaten either 30 minutes before sardines *or* three hours after sardines.

Note: you can use the following in moderation: fresh and dried herbs, salt and pepper, lemon, Bragg Liquid Aminos, ginger, garlic, scallions, onion.

Day six: fast—no food, only lemon water.

Note: after this day of fasting, reintroducing foods too soon will upset your stomach and ruin the effects of the diet.

Day seven: eat only brown rice, apples, and sardines. (See additional instructions for days four to five.)

Day eight: don't eat any animal protein except sardines, otherwise eat any foods from permitted foods category.

Days nine to ten: eat any foods from permitted foods category.

Bonus Cleansing Exercises: Working the Mind with the Body

The following exercises are all simple activities you can do to further cleanse your body, exercise your mental flexibility, and keep you from getting stuck mentally, physically, or spiritually. Every morning after you drink your lemon water, do these exercises to help your body and mind find connection, balance, and clarity. If your schedule doesn't allow for extra time in the morning, choose a time that works for you. See the checklist at the end of this step to help you plan your schedule.

Massage Your Abdomen

This will help push things through to clear your digestive system.

1. Sit somewhere comfortable and place your hand over your belly.

2. Gently massage in a circular motion, clockwise, for 90 sec-onds. That's it!

Exercise Your Pelvic Floor

This exercise will help increase fluidity and flexibility in one of the body's three diaphragms. When these parts are working well, they flex easily and are convex, or shaped like a smile, when at rest. Under stress however they can flatten and become rigid, disrupting the easy, natural flow we always want to have moving throughout our physical and psycho-spiritual terrains.

When people hear the word *diaphragm*, they tend to think about the thoracic diaphragm, the one in our abdominal area that expands and contracts, allowing us to breathe. However, the word actually refers to any separating membrane or structure, and there are two additional diaphragms in the body—the choroid plexus in the fourth ventricle of the brain and the pelvic diaphragm underneath the pelvis. To strengthen your pelvic floor, as you engage in your morning urination, think about controlling the flow.

1. Let the stream start flowing for a moment, then hold it, then let it go, then hold it.
2. Continue this way until you've emptied your bladder.

Exercise Your Eyes

Do you want to change your outlook? Has a thought or memory ever gotten stuck in your mind and you want to move past it? Start by moving your eyes. Your optic nerve is connected to your brain, so when you move your eyes, you move your brain. This is a great and simple way to change your perspective. It's best to do this exercise outside, but inside a spacious room will do. Just make sure not to do it while looking at any sort of screen.

1. Move your eyes at random in any and all directions. There's no magic pattern, just move them. If you have a cat, follow it with your eyes as it darts around the backyard. Or let your eyes follow a fly as it flits about.
2. Continue for 90 seconds, then stop and let your eyes rest for a moment before moving on to the next step.
3. Do the exercise again, but this time do it in conjunction with the tide breathing exercise on page 140 for added effect.

Exercise Your Visual Memory

Your eyes are the quickest way to connect your exterior world to your interior world, which is why this exercise will help foster connection between your body and mind. It will also help stretch and strengthen the choroid plexus diaphragm in the brain.

1. Walk by a shop window or a house on your street. After you've passed it, stop and ask yourself, "How many things did I see there?" In your mind, list as many things as you can.
2. Go back and see what you missed. Look around and try to find as many things as you can that you previously overlooked. It's not necessary to be exact or to score yourself on how many items you remember. So often we go through life with tunnel vision, so the aim here is to open up your vision so you can take this into the rest of your life and start seeing things more broadly.

THE COMPLETE CLARITY CLEANSE CHECKLIST

- ☐ Drink a large glass of lemon water.
- ☐ Do your bonus cleansing exercises.
- ☐ Massage your abdomen (90 seconds).
- ☐ Exercise your pelvic floor (90 seconds).
- ☐ Exercise your eyes (90 seconds).

Note: If you are doing these exercises in the morning, save the exercise for your visual memory for later in the day when you're out and about.

- ☐ Engage in PEW 12 or PEW 12-D (twelve minutes).
- ☐ Have a quiet time to recover from PEW 12 or PEW 12-D exercise (10 to 20 minutes minimum, or up to 90 minutes if needed).

Raising the Bar

When I was in high school and looking for a way to fit in, I gravitated toward athletics. Among the various sports I tried was pole vaulting, which uses a long flexible pole to propel a person over a high bar. It's an extremely difficult sport to learn, and the first time I tried it I fell directly on my face. The second and third times didn't go so well either. Only after I tried and tried again was I able to vault over the bar.

As you get ready to start your cleanse, you may feel a bit like I did as I held that pole in my hand for the first time and looked up at the high bar. This cleanse may seem like a lot to manage. You may be worried about the amount of negative energy you will bring up over the course of ten days. Or you might be concerned that you won't be able to do the IU Diet for this length of time.

The pursuit of clarity is a bit like psycho-spiritual pole vaulting. With each effort, we learn something about how to propel ourselves upward, even when we fall on our faces. Like with any sport, any discipline really, the combination of preparedness and practice helps us get better and better. Pretty soon we are clearing higher and higher bars.

As you embark on this cleanse, keep in mind that you have already prepared for this. We are now on step eleven of this process, and if you have worked through the previous steps, then you are ready for this. This doesn't mean there won't be obstacles or difficulties, but you now have the tools to handle such things. For example, if you find yourself encountering resistance, return to step five and ask questions about what you're feeling and why. If you find yourself feeling depleted, return to step ten and try some of the different methods for restoring your energy. In many ways this process for creating clarity is all about preparedness. It prepares you to handle whatever may come. So if you find yourself hitting a roadblock, remember to use what you've learned.

Clarity for Life

We have come a long way since the start of this process and our journey together is nearly complete. For this last step, let's take a look at how you can keep creating clarity in your life long after the last word in this book has been read.

The first thing to understand is that there's no end to the pursuit of clarity. As long as we are alive, we will continue to encounter circumstances that cause us to suffer, that are difficult to manage for one reason or another, or that leave us feeling cluttered and clogged. That is what this process is for, what this book is for. When something happens in your life, you can always come back to these pages to help you become unstuck, recover, and grow as a result of your experience.

It's like learning to ride a bike. Sometimes you'll have reason to ride, sometimes you won't, but once you've learned, you will always know how. It's a skill that will always be waiting for you whenever you need it, perhaps requiring just a little practice to help you get back into it. What you have learned in this book will always be there to help you get your life moving in the direction you want it to go, no matter what circumstances may be getting in your way.

It's also important to understand that you don't have to wait for trying times to make the pursuit of clarity a lifelong habit. You can decide to make cleansing, both physically and psycho-spiritually, a regular ritual, just like it is in many religions. You can decide to practice restoring yourself regularly by returning to the ideas and exercises in step ten as often as needed. As you'll read in the coming pages, you can practice having faith that things will turn out the way you want them to, no matter what lies ahead.

Clarity isn't easy. It requires effort and persistence. When I think about the labor required, I'm reminded of how E. E. Cummings in his letter "A Poet's Advice to Students" once described what it took to become a poet:

> *If, at the end of your first ten or fifteen years of fighting and working and feeling, you find you've written one line of one poem, you'll be very lucky indeed.*

Does that sound like a small payoff for so much effort? I don't think so, and neither did Cummings. As he wrote later in the same letter,

> *Does this sound dismal? It isn't.*
> *It's the most wonderful life on earth.*

"The most wonderful life on earth" is what I hope you will strive for through the pursuit of clarity. This final step is about learning to make clarity come alive in your life over the long term so that it lives beyond your experience of it in the pages of this book. I encourage you to make clarity a way of life for the rest of your life.

A POET'S ADVICE TO STUDENTS
E. E. CUMMINGS

A poet is somebody who feels, and who expresses his feeling through words.

This may sound easy. It isn't.

A lot of people think or believe or know they feel—but that's thinking or believing or knowing; not feeling. And poetry is feeling—not knowing or believing or thinking.

Almost anybody can learn to think or believe or know, but not a single human being can be taught to feel. Why? Because whenever you think or you believe or you know, you're a lot of other people: but the moment you feel, you're nobody-but-yourself.

To be nobody-but-yourself—in a world which is doing its best, night and day, to make you everybody else—means to fight the hardest battle which any human being can fight; and never stop fighting.

As for expressing nobody-but-yourself in words, that means working just a little harder than anybody who isn't a poet can possibly imagine. Why? Because nothing is quite as easy as using words like somebody else. We all of us do exactly this nearly all of the time—and whenever we do it, we are not poets.

If, at the end of your first ten or fifteen years of fighting and working and feeling, you find you've written one line of one poem, you'll be very lucky indeed.

And so my advice to all young people who wish to become poets is: do something easy, like learning how to blow up the world—unless you're not only willing, but glad, to feel and work and fight till you die.

Does this sound dismal? It isn't.
It's the most wonderful life on earth.
Or so I feel.

....

The Clarity Molecule

Over the past twelve years, since starting my medical practice, I have helped thousands of patients create more clarity in their lives and heal both physically and psycho-spiritually in the process. Years ago, I started noticing something curious about the way clarity changed people. I could obviously track certain changes based on what patients reported to me about how they were feeling, their levels of stress, their outlook for the future, and so on. At the same time, I was doing tests. The surprising thing I noticed when I looked first at my own lab results, then at those of my patients, was that clarity has a biological marker. The marker is the amount of oxytocin present in a person's bloodstream. Oxytocin is commonly known as the "love hormone" because it's released by both men and women during orgasm. It's also released by women during breastfeeding and childbirth, helping the mother bond with her baby. What I found time and time again was that when I measured the level of oxytocin present in my patients, for example before and after they did the Complete Clarity Cleanse, the results showed that their levels had gone up significantly.

I now measure oxytocin in my patients as a matter of course to use as an indicator of the progress we're making toward creating greater clarity for them. This is something you can do yourself by going to your primary physician and asking for a test. (Beforehand, you may want to check whether your insurance will cover this.) You will want to test before you start a new cleanse or before the next time you go through this process from beginning to end, then again after you've completed the cleanse or full process. When you compare the results, I can almost guarantee they will show your oxytocin levels higher than they were before.

My theory about the correlation between oxytocin and clarity has to do with love. Oxytocin is called the "love hormone," after all. When we clear ourselves of all the shoulds and shouldn'ts, the misinterpretations and the misidentifications, the preconceived judgments and limiting beliefs, we create space inside ourselves for something new. I believe we are all born with the seed of love already inside of us, resting there at the bottom of our cup. Love is our most natural state of being, but if our cup is crowded, cluttered, and clogged, it has no room to grow.

I once told this to a patient, who responded that she had learned the exact same thing from her agronomist father with respect to plants. All living things need room to grow, which is why in a garden you avoid planting things too close together. A potted plant needs to be moved to a larger vessel as it grows. Plants need space to stretch their roots and leaves in order to reach what Aristotle called *entelechy*, meaning to fully realize their potential. Entelechy is the natural force that allows a tiny acorn to change and grow into a towering tree. But if that seed doesn't have enough space as it attempts to grow, it will become stunted, sickly, and eventually die.

I have also found that once we have given the love inside us room to blossom, it becomes increasingly easier to maintain the feeling. Clarity leads to a boost in our oxytocin levels, oxytocin generates feelings of love, and the more love we feel the more clarity we will have. It's a self-supporting system, as long as we can keep the flow from being interrupted and provide the seed inside us with enough room to grow.

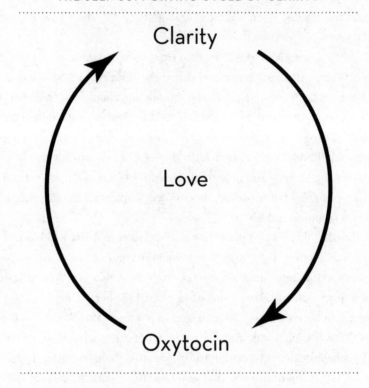

Clarity Requires Balance

So far we've talked mostly about how the flow of this self-supporting cycle is disrupted when we have too little clarity, but there is another side. There's such a thing as too much clarity. Like anything else in life, clarity is best when kept in balance.

Many people don't realize that the medications used to treat osteoporosis, a condition in which there's a thinning of bone in the body that can lead to stress fractures, came out of the space program.

When studying astronauts returning from space, scientists at NASA noticed that many of them would suffer bone fractures after seemingly innocuous incidents, like tripping over a curb. Further study of this curious trend revealed that astronauts' bones became thin and weakened due to the lack of gravity in space. They lost bone density because of the lack of pressure on their bones over an extended period.

When we have too much pressure in our lives, we become clogged. But too little pressure can be just as dangerous, leaving us open to injury. We need to strike a balance between bone being created and destroyed, between the judgmental and imaginal realms, and even between having too much "love hormone" in our systems or not enough. For clarity to be in balance, our oxytocin levels must also be in balance.

Taking drugs, overindulging in sex, or overdoing any number of stimulating activities results in a spike in oxytocin levels rather than a natural rise. This can cause someone to become obsessive, to chase the feeling that these activities inspire, which is a common characteristic of addiction.

How can anyone have too much love? Let's go back to the metaphor in this book where we described clarity in terms of a cup. We've learned that we need to empty the cup in order to make room for love to come in. But what happens if we generate the feeling of love in an inauthentic way, through taking drugs for example? Because we haven't taken the time to clean out our cup before letting in this love, it's just going to spill right over the top. If you increase the function without the structure to support it, you're going to overfill every time.

There are no shortcuts to clarity. No pill you can pop and no single act will create it over the long term. The high addicts experience is temporary because addiction is clarity without context. It's a pseudo clarity that simply won't last. This is why we've taken such care to work our way through an entire process that gets us ready for clarity in body, mind, and soul.

The American architect R. Buckminster Fuller came up with the term *tensegrity* to describe skeleton structures that evenly apply tension across their various parts so that each part operates with the maximum amount of efficiency and effectiveness. This is the kind of balance we're aiming for with clarity, evenly distributed tension across all aspects of our being. We want all parts of our lives, all at once, to open up to greater possibilities. Creating tensegrity for ourselves is how we create balance on a three-dimensional scale across the different aspects of our lives. If we don't keep up this tensegrity, sooner or later our clarity will come crashing down, just like it does with any addict when they come down from their high.

Clarity Requires Persistence: Persistence Is the Path to Faith

Living life in pursuit of clarity will require you to make some changes in your habits, the way you think, and how you handle situations and relationships. When we're trying to effect change in our lives, we're often told to have faith that it will happen. The problem with faith in this context is that it's intimidating. We're told we must believe in something unseen, unproven, and not previously experienced— with 100 percent of our being. We're also told that if we harbor one shred of doubt, even for a second, it's our fault that what we wanted didn't manifest in our lives. This just isn't true. So as you look toward a future filled with clarity, give yourself a break from this kind of pressure.

People who profess their faith too loudly are usually trying to convince themselves of the possibility of their desires or the validity of their beliefs. In other words they don't really have faith. They have doubts that they are trying to mask with showy displays of feigned faith. True faith is quiet and steadfast, and we exercise it in all sorts of different contexts. For example, you have faith that, when you get in your car tomorrow morning, the engine will start. It's not on your mind constantly, and you're not professing to everyone that this will happen. Because you've performed the proper upkeep on your car, and you're familiar with how your car works, you're certain it will be there for you in the morning when you need it. And it is practically every time.

We might say that faith isn't the result of blind belief but of understanding. When we understand what we must do to keep our car running smoothly, then we do it and the car performs as we desire. When we understand how the universal laws of manifestation work, then we can apply them in our lives with the expectation of manifestation. Why? Because we've done the work of studying them, applying them, and seeing their validity firsthand. When we understand and apply these spiritual laws, we don't have to try to believe in what's already self-evident.

The path to faith can be described as one of persistence. Continue visualizing your desire, preparing for its arrival, and living and feeling as if it's already arrived, and it will come. This is how the laws of manifestation work. Don't worry about worrying. Fear can be difficult to shake off sometimes, but this doesn't mean you're doing anything wrong. It just means you're human. You've learned how to deal with doubt and fear in this process. (See step six if you could use a reminder.) You can always return to the lessons in the book to get you back on track. Consistency is king. Soon you will find that you do indeed have that quiet assurance within you. You'll find that fear comes far less often, maybe even not at all. This is when you know you are close to manifestation and that the arrival of what you want is imminent. In this way faith isn't something you have, it's something you acquire through gaining understanding and doing the work.

We live in a universe where so-called reality is relative to the person experiencing it. We literally create our own realities based on our perceptions and what we hold to be true about ourselves and our world. It's that simple. While there may be people in your life who mean well when they try to prevent you from being disappointed when you don't get what you want, they do so based on their versions of reality, not yours. You don't have to accept anyone else's version of reality.

For decades it was thought that a human couldn't run a mile in under four minutes. This limit on the capacity of the human body was accepted reality because no one had ever surpassed it. Fortunately this reality wasn't something that Roger Bannister believed in when, in 1954, he ran the first under-four-minute mile. His achievement then changed reality for others. Less than two months later, John Landy beat the four-minute mark, and by the end of 1957 fourteen other runners had as well. This is but one example, but I could give you countless others showing that reality is most certainly relative.

The antidote to limits is to keep cultivating your faith and consciously creating your own experience. As you do, it's important not to confuse faith with hope. Hope is a pessimist looking optimistically at things. Hope says, "Well, things probably aren't going to work out, but it would be nice if they did." Being hopeful is wanting the best but planning for the worst. Hope believes that there are forces greater than us that usually win. Hope is rooted in a feeling of lack or need. The feeling of need can only send out one signal, the frequency of need, which keeps us right on needing and never having what we want.

Faith on the other hand is believing you already have within you everything you need to achieve clarity. You don't have to buy anything or acquire anything. You just have to do the work. Continue to work this process and have faith in the outcome, and you will get there. You will have the life you always wanted.

EXERCISE:
Defining Reality Meditation

The following meditation will help you cultivate faith and define the reality you desire. Ideally this meditation should be read aloud, so find a quiet place where you can speak the words to yourself. Repeat them if you feel inspired to do so:

Faith is the natural byproduct of understanding and action. I don't need to have faith at the beginning of my journey as I move toward the manifestation of my desire. What I must have is a thorough understanding of how and why the universal laws of manifestation work. When I understand this process, I can put it into action. If I am consistent in my application of these laws, faith will be cultivated within my consciousness and arise as the result of what I'm doing.

Blind belief only leads to disappointment. Instead I will commit to learning all I can, then put what I've learned into practice with the full expectation of its effectiveness. I will not judge myself for moments of worry, doubt, or fear, but will continue in my work because I know that persistence is the path to faith and the realization of my desire. Just as surely as the law of gravity works every time the principle is applied, I know that the laws of manifestation are equally immutable. Therefore I remain as consistent as I can possibly be in thought and action, letting negative energy and fear pass through me as my manifestation draws closer and becomes imminent. When my manifestation arrives, there will be no need for me to try to believe in anything. I will know the law works. I will have absolute faith because the reality of the power of the law will have made itself known to me in a physical way.

I cultivate the quiet, steadfast assurance of faith within myself by creating a manifestation plan. Merely understanding universal law isn't enough to manifest my desire. I must put these principles into action. Therefore I love myself enough to commit to a daily practice of these activities and make them a top priority in my schedule. I don't need to believe anything at the outset of this journey, but to manifest my desire I must be consistent in my actions. Even though I may not see any change in the physical circumstances of my life or feel any different, I will continue on, knowing that change is indeed happening at the level of my consciousness. At the right time, I will experience the peaceful confidence that my desire is at hand, the faith that what I want is already here, and that is when my goal will be realized.

I surround myself with those who help support my faith-building efforts and move away from those who don't, even if their doubtful or fearful notions come out of genuine concern for me. These won't help me cultivate my faith. I know that reality is relative to the person experiencing it and their level of consciousness. I will not allow others' ideas about what reality is affect my faith and what I know is possible for me. I create my own reality through the content of my consciousness, and I place the fullness of my attention on the cultivation of faith that will manifest it in the way I have chosen.

Make Clarity an Active Process

Clarity is something you can use anytime something unexpected comes up in your life and knocks you off course. Responding to an issue is a good use of the tools in this book, but it's also a passive use. It's like waiting for the rain to come in order to take a shower. The alternative is to take your psycho-spiritual hygiene into your own hands and actively look for areas of your life to clean up.

In his book *People of the Lie*, psychiatrist M. Scott Peck describes an experience where he was sitting in a train station with his wife. As they waited for their train to come, he looked around and wondered why there was so much trash strewn about. As he continued looking, he realized what surely contributed to the clutter, the fact that throughout the entire station he couldn't see a single trash can.

Just because there are no trash cans doesn't mean that people don't make trash. This is something to think about as you move forward and pursue a life of clarity. You now have the tools to properly dispose of your emotional trash, but what happened before you had those tools? Your inner terrain probably looked like the floor of that train station, strewn with refuse because you didn't have a proper place to dispose of it. This is why, when you want to find opportunities to actively bring more clarity into your life, the best place to look is in your past.

This approach is similar to the "make amends" steps of Alcoholics Anonymous. These steps require alcoholics to look back at their lives, identify the people they've harmed as a result of their alcohol addiction, and do something to make amends to them. In much the same way, you can actively look for opportunities to bring deeper clarity to past events in your life.

I did this recently to clear the residue from an upsetting and embarrassing moment in my college career. My parents never went to college, so my brother and I were the first in our family to go. As a result, I felt an enormous amount of pressure to succeed. In a singular moment of weakness, I chose to cheat on a chemistry exam and got caught. Fortunately for me, the administration gave me another chance rather than kick me out of their program. I learned some important lessons from the experience, but the pain and humiliation have always lingered. As a result, I recently attempted to recontextualize and bring more clarity to the experience by writing my alma mater a letter. (See sidebar.)

In the letter, I explained what had happened to me and suggested that the pressure I felt was and still is common among college students. As a result, I proposed that the university start a new program of lectures that would feature speakers from a wide variety of professional sectors including medicine, science, literature, business, entertainment, and education with the intention of providing students with a broader perspective on life, as well as direction and inspiration about what's really important as they prepare to make their way in the world. It's the kind of guidance I needed back then and I believe many others could benefit from it as well.

As a result of that letter, the university is now creating a program like the one I proposed, funded by an endowment named after my late brother and all the professors and administrators who were helpful to me during that difficult time in my life, including the one who caught me cheating! You can do something similar in your own life by looking for creative ways to address negative experiences in your past. My advice would be to start large and go small. I call this the macro-to-microcosm approach, which means starting with the moments that have the potential to make the greatest impact by bringing clarity to them. Another way of approaching this is to imagine yourself at the age of 100 looking back on your life, then ask yourself, "What would I most regret leaving unresolved or not clarified?" That's where you should start. You may be surprised how much satisfaction you get out of turning your most difficult moments into opportunities to make a big impact.

To: Soraya M. Coley, President
California State Polytechnic University, Pomona
Dear President Coley:

I am a proud graduate of Cal Poly, Class of 1994. In the years since graduation, my life as a physician has been filled with its share of blessings. Like many people, I have reflected on the previous decades and wondered whether that young, struggling student could have had any idea where his life would be in the year 2016, particularly considering the challenges he faced at the time. Fortunately for me, the compassion and insight of several outstanding Cal Poly faculty members not only helped me navigate those challenges, but played an integral role in shaping how I live my life today.

My family immigrated to the U.S. from Iran when I was twelve. Culture shock doesn't begin to describe how difficult the transition was for me. I was still struggling with the culture and language when I reached Cal Poly six years later. My difficulties were compounded by the fact that my younger brother, Mehrdad, and I were the first two people in our family to go to college. Naturally, our family was proud, but where there is great pride, there is even greater expectation. The pressure to succeed created a burden of stress that was virtually unbearable.

Ultimately, this stress led me to make the biggest mistake of my academic career. In a singular moment of weakness, I chose to cheat on a chemistry exam. Fortunately, I was caught. Even though I suffered crushing humiliation, the blessing was that I could begin to free myself from my unhealthy drive to achieve. I will forever be grateful for the compassionate and nonjudgmental way in which then Vice President of Academic Affairs, Dr. Robert Naples, and my advisor, Dr. Brigitte Goehler, handled the matter and brought peace and perspective back into my life.

I'm sure I wasn't the only student back then living under a great deal of pressure from a combination of cultural, familial, academic, and personal stresses. I also think it's fair to assume that many students today face the same challenges. For this reason, I would like to make a proposal to help these students through the creation of an ongoing lecture series.

This series would feature speakers from a wide variety of professional sectors. The intention is to provide students with a broader perspective on life, as well as direction and inspiration about what's really important as they prepare to make their way in the world. Lecturers would discuss the kind of subjects we don't usually get graded on, like developing a sense of maturity and responsibility, living ethically and with compassion, cultivating self-confidence, and finding the courage to live your passion. I believe the purpose of higher education isn't just to prepare graduates for careers, but to produce conscientious adults who understand themselves and how to interact with the world so they can contribute to making it a better place. Supplementing the existing excellent curriculum with this kind of lecture series would help create a truly integrated experience that not only shapes the students' minds, but also feeds their souls.

If this proposal should meet with your approval, it would mean a great deal to me if you would consider naming the endowment after those teachers and administrators who helped shape my character and future. I thank you for your consideration and look forward to working with you to advocate for students in this essential way.

In appreciation,
Dr. Habib Sadeghi

The Impact of Clarity on a Global Scale

As a final word, I would like to inspire you to continue your path toward greater and greater clarity by suggesting an even larger purpose. Achieving clarity isn't only important on a personal level, it's essential on a global scale. Everyone's personal happiness matters because we live in a world that's governed by and made up entirely of energy. Quantum physics has shown us that inside the smallest bit of physical matter we know, the atom, there is largely open space. In fact, it's 99.999 percent open space. There's nothing there except a handful of subatomic particles floating like dust in the air. Matter doesn't come from matter. It comes from energy vibrating at an infinite number of different frequencies.

This means every human being is vibrating at a specific frequency that perfectly matches his or her combination of thoughts and feelings. As energetic beings, we're not islands unto ourselves. We're mixing and sharing frequencies every moment of our lives with every other human on the planet. Every day, our personal energetic note combines with the frequencies from 7.3 billion people to create a collective vibration that relates to the level of consciousness of the human race as a whole. I think it's fair to say that when you look at the state of our physical world today, our energetic symphony is way off-key. I believe this is because far too many people are emitting negative frequencies grounded in base emotions like fear, hatred, resentment, greed, doubt, and hopelessness. Our mistake has been to try to save the world by acting on physical circumstances alone. This is where you and I come in.

Paul J. Zak, a professor of economic psychology at Claremont Graduate University and the author of *The Moral Molecule*, has been interested in the hormone oxytocin much like I have, but for somewhat different reasons. He calls oxytocin "the moral molecule" because his research suggests it has a profound effect on our social behavior. Oxytocin, he contends, is present when we trust one another. This could mean trusting our intimate partner, someone we're doing a business deal with, or a stranger. What's more, he believes that trust is the single most important factor in determining how well a society works as a whole. Zak writes in his book, "I spent more than a year demonstrating that the level of trust in a society is the single most powerful determinant of whether that society prospers or remains mired in poverty. Being able to enforce contracts, being able to rely on others to deliver what they promise and not cheat or steal, is a more powerful factor in a country's economic development than education, access to resources—anything."

We are inspired to produce oxytocin because of our interactions with one another, such as when we feel love for a partner or child, or when we trust someone in our community. Trust isn't required when we're alone. It's required when people interact with one another. Clarity also shows up through our interactions with others. We notice that we have clarity or that we are clogged when we encounter people in our lives and respond to them either based on what's happening in the moment (clarity) or based on past experiences that have led us to harbor preconceived judgments, misinterpretations, or limiting beliefs (a lack of clarity). Love, trust, and clarity don't exist in a vacuum. They are part of the common terrain we share with others, affecting and affected by every person we come into contact with.

For me this means we don't have to travel halfway around the world to help starving children, end wars, or heal the sick. "Be the change you want to see in the world," as many mystics say. We can start healing the world by healing ourselves. Each time one more person achieves clarity and begins living authentically, this shift in consciousness significantly impacts the energetic frequency, the oxytocin level, and the consciousness level of the entire human race. Like ripples on a lake or currents in an ocean, the higher vibrations fan out across the globe and affect every living person.

This brings the human race closer to clarity as a whole and all the wonderful benefits that come with it, like peace, prosperity, healthy relationships, and love. This is how important each one of us is to the entire world. I believe it's why we're here on this planet—to help heal it by first healing ourselves. It's time to awaken our personal power and manifest a world that's waiting for all of us. We can get there if we all follow the path to clarity.

CLARITY FOR LIFE—PRACTICING GOOD PSYCHO-SPIRITUAL HYGIENE

The following is a list of things you can do to make creating clarity a habit you engage in for the rest of your life.

- *Make the ten-day Intentional Unsaturation Diet an annual event:* I recommend doing it at the beginning of a transitional season, either spring or fall. Transitions are the times in our lives when we are most likely to become clogged and could do with a bit of spring-cleaning, so to speak. Most illnesses, including cancers, come about in the spring or fall for this reason. They are also likely to arise at times of transition in our lives: after a divorce, when a loved one has died, and so on. Cleansing can help us through times of transition.
- *Return to the PEW 12 exercises on a regular basis, particularly when you're going through a trying time in your life:* PEW 12 is a quick and easy enough exercise that you could even make it part of your morning ritual, as a means of practicing good emotional hygiene on a

regular basis. Each morning you might get up, brush your teeth, and sit down for twelve minutes to write in your notebook before starting your day. If every day seems like too much, aim to do it three to five days a week.

- *Distance yourself from people who tell you that you can't have the things in your life you believe clarity will bring:* By this I mean people who urge you to be "realistic" about your odds of recovering from illness, getting that coveted job, having a relationship that's truly fulfilling, or achieving whatever it is you truly desire.

- *Search out opportunities to make clarity an active rather than a passive process:* We can take our psycho-spiritual hygiene into our own hands by looking for creative ways to address negative past experiences and bring deeper clarity to them. As we do, I suggest starting with what will have the greatest impact on your life—the macro-to-microcosm approach I talked about earlier. Of course, as we call up difficult memories from our past, we always need to have compassion for ourselves and remember that we did the best we could based on what we knew at the time.

- *Join the Love Button Global Movement:* By creating clarity, we open up space inside ourselves where love can come rushing in, love that will enhance our own lives and that we can share with others to create a better world. The Love Button Global Movement (LoveButton.org) was established to educate and empower people to transform their communities through loving acts of kindness. By joining, you can find opportunities to share love with people all over the planet and make this world a better place to live for all of us.

Everything Is Possible, or a Stem Cell Way of Being

You have probably heard of stem cells. In the United States stem cells have been the focus of a high-profile political battle over whether they should be harvested from embryos for medical purposes. The drama of that battle has overshadowed what stem cells really are and why they are so remarkable.

A stem cell is an unspecialized cell that's pluripotent, which means it has the potential to be all kinds of different things. In other words, a stem cell is a cell that has yet to be given a task or definition. If you insert a stem cell into a brain, it becomes a neuron. If you insert it into a toenail, it becomes part of the toenail. If you insert it into a heart, it learns to work with the other heart cells to pump blood through the body. A stem cell becomes whatever is around it.

True clarity is a stem cell way of being. It happens as a result of clearing out all the residue of past experiences that create and reinforce limiting beliefs, preconceived judgments, and misperceptions that tell us how things are or how they should or shouldn't be. When the residue is cleared away, what we're left with is a state of infinite possibilities, which can create a more conducive terrain for healing, fulfillment, and love. In the context of absolute clarity, we have the potential to create whatever we want. As a Buddhist quote says, "Being nothing, you are everything."

Clarity is how I define God, or whatever we want to call our Higher Power. God is the stem cell, the ultimate clarity, the thing of infinite possibilities. Many think of themselves as a body that houses a soul. I think of humanity in a different way. I think we are all divine souls having a human experience here on earth.

Recall that I shared with you how, back when I thought I was going to die from cancer, my friend and mentor Gary gave me a gold South African Krugerrand to help me remember that "love is that gold you keep inside you." It symbolized for me my golden soul, the source of the voice I heard at a crucial point in my life telling me not to accept my doctor's invasive treatment plan but instead trust that I could find a better way to heal. That moment made all the difference in my life. It was the beginning of a process that helped me come to understand this thing I call clarity. That in turn inspired me to start a medical practice so I could teach others about clarity, which in due course led me here to this book so I could show even more people what it means to live a life of clarity.

I have kept this gold coin in my wallet ever since. It sits alongside another coin I received on the journey that followed, when I took a year off medical school to travel and learn more about different healing techniques in places like Mexico, India, and Germany. While I was in Mexico, I met a *curandero*, a native healer who listened to me talk about how full of doubt I was about choosing to forgo most of my doctor's treatment plan and how I was feeling less than whole as a result of the surgery I'd undergone to remove the testicle where the cancer had been found. "A real man has two," I kept telling this healer. As a result, he gave me a 1932 Mexican peso that was meant as a bit of a joke and also a form of reassurance. He told me with a smile that it was "*un peso*" to represent my "one ball," but it was also meant as a symbol of the oneness, the wholeness that I still embodied. The silver coin was dark and tarnished but its value was undiminished because of its scarred surface. He was telling me in his own good-natured way that I was still a man and always would be in this life, no matter what might happen to alter my physical appearance.

In the years since then, I have kept those two coins in my wallet, where no one sees them but me. One is shiny and gold, the other tarnished silver, and I pull them out from time to time to provide myself with a visual representation of the idea that we are all golden souls having a human experience.

As our divine souls make our way through this life, we are bound by the laws of the world in which we live and can never quite attain absolute clarity. We will get battered and tarnished along the way, which is simply part of being human, but there's still so much power and beauty in striving for an infinite state of being.

The more we reach for clarity, the more space we create in our consciousness. The more space we create, the more room there is inside us for love to expand and grow. Love is a natural state of being, the divine state of being. When we empty ourselves of all the clutter and muck we have been needlessly carrying around with us from experience to experience, love naturally grows in the space we have created. As it says in the Bible (I John 4:8 NIV), "Whoever does not love does not know God, because God is love."

This is what I want you to think about as you finish this process and continue your journey toward clarity on your own. Too often people resign themselves to living lives that aren't worthy of them because they don't think they can have something better. I believe every one of us can have more, can *be* more. There are numerous statements in the Bible that assure us God is willing to give us more if we only ask for it, such as, "Ask, and it will be given to you; seek and you will find; knock and the door will be opened to you" (Matthew 7:7 NIV).

You don't have to believe in any organized religion, or even God for that matter, in order to understand the possibilities inherent in creating clarity for yourself. You can choose instead to believe in the stem cell, the basic building block of all humanity, which is where you and every one of us started. Too many of us lose out on a great relationship, a fulfilling job, a beautiful experience, a full and wonderful life because we don't ask for it. We don't ask because we don't believe we can have it.

There are no shortcuts to living the life you've always wanted to live, to being the person you've always wanted to be. You have to start by believing. You have to believe, you have to ask, and you have to do the work, so that when you ask for what you want you will feel deserving of it. There's a difference between asking for tea with your cup held tightly to your breast so that it's difficult for the pourer to reach it and asking with your arm outstretched, holding your empty cup out in an open gesture of receiving.

Young children instinctively ask openly and without shame, embarrassment, fear, or doubt for what they want. They do this because they aren't yet clogged. It isn't until we grow older and learn to put limits on ourselves that we stop asking. In a way, the process of creating clarity takes us backward to our child selves who were unafraid to ask, who believed we could be whatever we wanted to be, who never even thought to ask the question, "Am I worthy of this?" because the answer was clear. Of course we are worthy.

If we try and keep trying, we may be able to travel back further than this, to what we were before our child selves came into the world, to that stem cell way of being that was our starting place—a state of infinite potential. This is what I believe is possible for you. It's what I believe is possible for all of us.

Blessings on your journey.

STEM CELL WAY OF BEING

There is a reason for me to keep coming here; here, where the sun shines warmly, just right.

Here, where there is a magic already pre-Sent and everything possibly possible is already, Here.

Here, where as I arrive unto the greeting of a funnel, all scripted differentiations, specializations, judgments, misunderstandings, misinterpretations and the quickly crystallized misidentifications peel off with Ease & Grace.

Here, where time after time, I'm left with the Stem Cell of Loving to find my way Home.

Here, where Acceptance does not equate Agreement to being a certain way.

Here, where God greets me smiling by the door.

—Dr. Habib Sadeghi
July 24, 2016
Santa Monica, California

Appendix

Glossary
Ten-Day Intentional Unsaturation Diet Plan
IU Diet Recipes from the Goop Test Kitchen
The "Being" List
Meditation Moments

Glossary

anabolism: The process of building something up.

caesura: Any cut or crisis that affords us an opportunity to learn and grow, to move forward in conscious evolution.

catabolism: The process of breaking something down.

emotional armoring: A means of avoiding our emotions or their cause by creating blocks against them.

emotional posturing: A means of repressing our emotions by pretending our lives or our situations are different/better than they actually are.

entelechy: The vital force that encourages a thing to fully realize its potential.

imaginal realm: The internal world, where we encounter the invisible and abstract—our thoughts, feelings, memories, and ideas.

judgmental realm: The external world, where we encounter things that are visible and concrete; also where we project our judgments of the things we encounter.

judgments, conscious: Judgments based on a clear view of the information we have in front of us, rather than on past experiences or preconceived ideas.

judgments, preconceived: Judgments that are based on past experiences rather than a full understanding and processing of the situation that is unfolding in front of us.

negative capability: Concept put forth by the English Romantic poet John Keats, which describes a person's ability to sit with the mystery of life and trust the process, even when they don't know how things will turn out.

projection: An outward manifestation or our inner reality.

psychosomatic: From the ancient Greek *psycho*, meaning mind, and *soma*, meaning body. Healers at the time believed that all illness was a mind-body event, requiring treatment on both fronts.

psycho-spiritual: A combination of the psychological and spiritual.

psycho-spiritual hygiene: The practice of regularly cleaning out the negative energy from our minds and spirits.

self-doubt, healthy: The ability to accept a situation as it is without needing to fill in all the blanks or know all the answers. It's about knowing that we don't know everything and allowing this to be okay as we move forward.

self-doubt, unhealthy: To have doubts about ourselves and our circumstances that compel us to unconsciously make choices that don't serve us.

self-knowledge: Being able to see ourselves and the situations in our lives clearly and without judgment.

self-parent: The process, usually taught to us by our parents, of processing or digesting our emotions by holding or containing them long enough to break them down, taking what we can use from them and discarding the rest.

stem cell: An unspecialized, pluripotent cell, which means it has the potential to be all kinds of different things depending on the context it's placed in.

tensegrity: A term borrowed from American architect R. Buckminster Fuller, who used it to describe skeleton structures that evenly apply tension across their various parts so that each part operates with the maximum amount of efficiency and effectiveness. In the context of this book, tensegrity is the kind of three-dimensional balance we're aiming for by creating clarity in our bodies, minds, and spirits all at once.

terrain: The collective impact of all the defining factors and decisions made about an environment in the past and present that affect how it performs in the present. A terrain can be physical, like a plot of land or your body, or it can be nonphysical, like your consciousness or the collective consciousness of a family, community, or even the entire world.

Ten-Day Intentional Unsaturation Diet Plan

FOOD CATEGORIES	DAY OF DIET
Animal Protein:	**Day 1:**
All poultry, all fish and shellfish, egg whites	Anything from any category
Vegetables:	**Day 2:**
All vegetables including nightshades and herbs	Anything from any category
Fruits:	**Day 3:**
All fresh and unsweetened frozen fruit, no dried fruit	Avoid animal protein category Anything from all other categories
Apples:	**Day 4:**
Only fresh pink or red; eat only when they've turned brown being exposed to air	Only brown rice, apples, and sardines Can use in moderation to dress these foods: fresh from or dried herbs, salt and pepper, lemon, Bragg Aminos, ginger, garlic, scallions, onion

Sardines:	**Day 5:**
Canned (packed in olive oil) or fresh	Only brown rice, apples, and sardines Same options to dress foods as day 4
Brown Rice:	**Day 6:**
All kinds in moderation (1–2 cups per day total)	Fast: no food; drink only lemon water
	Day 7:
	Only brown rice, apples, and sardines Same options to dress foods as day 4
	Day 8:
	Avoid animal protein category Anything from all other categories
	Day 9:
	Anything from any category
	Day 10:
	Anything from any category

IU Diet Recipes from the Goop Test Kitchen

Many thanks to Gwyneth Paltrow and the talented people at goop who crafted these wonderful recipes to work with the IU Diet.

All recipes will yield one serving unless otherwise noted.

....

"The 10 days on the IU Diet were challenging, transforming, and uplifting. It's something I will return to yearly for healing and a deep reset."   —Gwyneth Paltrow

....

Fennel and Seared Shrimp Salad—days 1, 2, 9, 10
Clean Veggie Slaw—days 1–3, 8–10
Arugula and Watermelon Radish Salad—days 1–3, 8–10
Sweet Potato Soup—days 1–3, 8–10
Bagna Cauda Platter—days 1–3, 8–10
Rice Porridge—days 1–5, 7–10
Fried Brown Rice—days 1–5, 7–10
Caramelized Onions with Rice and Sardines—days 1–5, 7–10
Grilled Vegetable and Chicken Salad with Pistou—days 1, 2, 9, 10
Pistou—days 1–5, 7–10
Eggplant Parmesan—days 1–3, 8–10

Clean Salmon Burgers—days 1, 2, 9, 10

Roasted Sunchokes and Cauliflower with Caper Sauce—days 1–3, 8–10

Grilled Sardines—days 1–5, 7–10

Pan-Seared Sardines with Capers and Lemon—days 1–5, 7–10

Poached Sardines with Lemon and Chili—days 1–5, 7–10

Clean Bok Choy—days 1–3, 8–10

Roasted Sweet Potato Dessert—days 1–3, 8–10

Clean Veggie Chips—days 1–3, 8–10

Fennel and Seared Shrimp Salad

5 shrimp, peeled and deveined

3 tablespoons olive oil

Sea salt and cracked pepper to taste

½ cup chopped romaine

½ cup chopped endive

½ cup chopped radicchio

1 tablespoon each chopped chives, cilantro, basil, and mint

1 small fennel bulb, finely sliced

Juice of 1 large Meyer lemon

½ avocado, sliced

Heat a small sauté pan over medium-high heat, toss the shrimp with a teaspoon of olive oil, salt and pepper, and sear until nicely browned on each side and cooked through (about 6 minutes total).

Meanwhile, combine the romaine, endive, radicchio, fresh herbs, and sliced fennel in a bowl. Toss with lemon juice, olive oil, salt and pepper, and adjust seasoning as needed.

Plate the salad, garnish with seared shrimp and sliced avocado, and finish with cracked black pepper and a little sea salt.

Clean Veggie Slaw

. . . .

FOR THE DRESSING:
Zest and juice of ½ Meyer lemon
Zest and juice of ½ lime
Zest and juice of 1 small orange or tangerine
1 tablespoon finely minced red chili
3 tablespoons olive oil
Generous pinch of salt

FOR THE SLAW:
2 scallions, thinly sliced
1 cup finely sliced Napa cabbage
1 cup finely sliced red cabbage
1 large or 2 small carrots, peeled and grated
½ red bell pepper, thinly sliced
⅓ cup chopped cilantro

In a large bowl, whisk together the dressing ingredients.

Add the slaw ingredients, and toss to evenly coat. Taste for seasoning and add more salt if necessary.

Arugula and Watermelon Radish Salad

. . . .

1 roasted beet, peeled and cut into large dice
2 roasted carrots, cut into bite-sized pieces
½ avocado, diced
1 large handful arugula
¼ cup chopped cilantro
1 tablespoon lemon juice
3 tablespoons olive oil
Salt and pepper

Combine all ingredients in a bowl.

Sweet Potato Soup

. . . .

2 tablespoons olive oil
½ medium onion, diced
2 medium leeks, diced
1 large carrot, diced
2 celery stalks, diced
3 garlic cloves, peeled and minced
1 large and 1 small sweet potato, peeled and cut into 1-inch
    chunks
2 rosemary sprigs
1 bay leaf
6 cups water
Salt
Juice of ½ lemon

Heat olive oil in a Dutch oven or saucepan over medium-high heat, then add onion and leek and sauté for 5 minutes. Add carrot, celery, and garlic, and cook another 5 minutes. Add sweet potato, rosemary, bay leaf, water, and a couple large pinches of salt.

Bring to a boil, reduce heat to simmer, and cook for 20–30 minutes, or until sweet potato pieces are tender.

Blend, add lemon juice, and adjust seasoning as needed.

Garnish with cracked pepper, chili flake, and sea salt.

Bagna Cauda Platter

. . . .

FOR THE BAGNA CAUDA:
1 garlic clove, minced
¼ cup olive oil

4 anchovies, chopped
Pinch chili flakes
10 grinds black pepper
Zest and juice of ½ lemon

FOR CRUDITÉ:
Any crudité you like, such as...
  1 head endive, separated into leaves
  ½ small head radicchio, cut into large pieces
  1 small head fennel, cut into large pieces
  8 asparagus spears, quickly blanched and cut in half
  6 Brussels sprouts, separated into individual leaves

Combine first five ingredients for the bagna cauda in a small saucepan over medium-low heat. Cook, stirring constantly with a wooden spoon, until the anchovies have melted and the garlic is fragrant, but not burned. Add lemon zest and juice, and taste for seasoning.

Transfer the warm dip to a bowl and serve with assorted crudité.

Rice Porridge

  1 cup short-grain brown rice
  7 cups water
  1 vanilla pod, scraped
  1 large pinch Maldon sea salt
  ½ teaspoon cinnamon
  ⅛ teaspoon nutmeg
  ⅛ teaspoon cardamom

Combine all ingredients in a slow cooker and cook on "low" setting (7 or 8 hours).

Note: For a savory variation, add crushed garlic and sliced ginger instead of vanilla and spices, and garnish with Bragg Liquid Aminos and sliced scallions.

Fried Brown Rice

2 tablespoons olive oil
1 cup cooked brown rice
1 small garlic clove, minced
1 teaspoon finely minced ginger
2 scallions, thinly sliced
1 tablespoon Bragg Liquid Aminos

Heat olive oil in a large nonstick pan over medium-high heat. When the oil is hot but not smoking, add the cooked rice, garlic, and ginger and mix with a wooden spoon to combine.

Continue to cook for 3 to 5 minutes, stirring occasionally, then add the scallions and Bragg. Taste for seasoning and add salt if necessary.

Caramelized Onions with Rice and Sardines

3 tablespoons olive oil
1 medium yellow onion, thinly sliced
Salt and pepper
½ cup cooked brown rice
½ can sardines packed in olive oil, drained and broken into bite-
    sized pieces

Heat the oil in a large sauté pan over medium heat.

Add sliced onion, a generous pinch of salt, and a few grinds of black pepper.

Reduce the heat to low, cover the pan, and allow the onions to slow cook for 30 minutes, until meltingly tender and very sweet.

Turn the heat up to medium, add cooked rice and sardines to the pan, stir with a wooden spoon, and cook for a couple of minutes, just to warm everything through.

Grilled Vegetable and Chicken Salad with Pistou

1 chicken breast, pounded into a thin cutlet

Olive oil

Salt and pepper

4 large asparagus spears

3 scallions

5 pieces Broccolini, quickly blanched in salted water

1 Meyer lemon

2 tablespoons pistou, plus more for serving (recipe follows)

Heat a grill pan over medium-high heat and season the chicken cutlet with olive oil, salt, and pepper. Grill chicken for about 3 minutes per side (depending on thickness) or until cooked through with nice grill marks. Remove to a plate to rest.

Meanwhile, toss the asparagus, scallions, and blanched Broccolini with 1 tablespoon olive oil and season with salt and pepper. Grill these for about 5 minutes, or until charred and tender.

Cut the chicken and veggies into bite-sized pieces and toss with the juice of ½ Meyer lemon and 2 tablespoons pistou.

Serve with extra lemon wedges and pistou on the side.

Pistou

⅔ cup chopped basil
⅓ cup arugula or parsley leaves
1 small garlic clove, roughly chopped
2 teaspoons lemon zest
½ teaspoon salt
½ cup olive oil

Combine all ingredients in a blender or food processor. Blend until smooth.

Note: Use pistou in the Eggplant Parmesan, Grilled Vegetable and Chicken Salad, and Grilled Sardines recipes.

Eggplant Parmesan

This recipe has a lot of components, but once the tomatoes are roasted, it is fairly quick to put together. You can also make the slow-roasted tomatoes, the pistou, and the eggplant in advance.

Serves 2

FOR THE SLOW-ROASTED TOMATOES:
6 organic vine-ripened tomatoes, cut in half horizontally
1 tablespoon olive oil

FOR THE EGGPLANT:
1 medium eggplant
Salt and pepper
¼ cup olive oil

FOR THE SALAD:
1 large handful arugula
8 cherry tomatoes, sliced in half
Juice of ½ lemon
2 tablespoons olive oil
Salt and pepper

Begin by roasting the tomatoes. Preheat oven to 275 degrees, toss halved tomatoes with olive oil, and arrange cut-side up in a small roasting tray.

Roast tomatoes in the oven for 2 hours.

While the tomatoes roast, make the pistou. (See pistou recipe, page 256.)

Cut the eggplant into 1-inch slices, season generously with salt and pepper, and drizzle with olive oil. Heat a grill pan over medium-high heat and grill until tender (about 5 minutes per side).

Just before serving, combine all salad ingredients in a large bowl and toss.

Divide arugula salad between two plates, then layer 1 slice of eggplant and top with 1 tablespoon pistou and two roasted tomato halves. Repeat twice more layering eggplant, pistou, and roasted tomatoes.

Clean Salmon Burgers

Makes 6 patties
1 ½ pounds salmon, skin removed and cut into 1-inch pieces
4 scallions, sliced
1 garlic clove, peeled and crushed
⅓ cup roughly chopped cilantro
1 small red chili, deseeded and chopped
1 2-inch piece fresh ginger, peeled and roughly chopped

2 tablespoons Bragg Liquid Aminos
½ teaspoon salt

Place salmon pieces in the freezer for about 10 minutes, until very cold but not frozen. In batches, add the salmon to a food processor and pulse until it is well minced but before it becomes a paste, about 10 pulses per batch.

Remove the salmon to a large bowl and blend the remaining ingredients in the food processor until very smooth, about one minute. Add to the bowl with the salmon, mix well, cover, and refrigerate overnight.

To cook, place a grill pan over medium-high heat. Form the salmon mixture into 6 patties, and when the pan is hot but not smoking, grill burgers for 3 minutes on each side.

Roasted Sunchokes and Cauliflower with Caper Sauce

6 sunchokes, scrubbed and cut into bite-sized pieces if large
2 tablespoons olive oil
3 whole, skin-on garlic cloves
1 pinch chili flakes
1 sprig rosemary
Salt and pepper
1 small head cauliflower, cut into florets

FOR THE SAUCE:
3 tablespoons olive oil
¼ cup capers, drained well
1 anchovy fillet, finely chopped
1 garlic clove, minced
1 teaspoon grated lemon zest

Heat oven to 400 degrees.

Toss sunchokes on a baking sheet with olive oil, garlic cloves, chili flakes, and rosemary sprig and season generously with salt and pepper. Roast for 40 minutes, until very crispy. Add cauliflower to the baking sheet and continue to roast for 15–20 minutes or until cauliflower is cooked through and beginning to brown.

Just before the veggies are ready, make the sauce. Heat the olive oil in small sauté pan over medium heat. When the oil is hot but not smoking, add the capers and fry for 2–3 minutes, until they begin to crisp up. Add anchovy, minced garlic, and lemon zest and turn down the heat to medium low and continue to cook for a few more minutes, or until the anchovy is melted and the garlic is fragrant but not burned.

To serve, pour the sauce over the roasted veggies.

Grilled Sardines

3 whole sardines scaled, gutted, and deboned
Zest of 1 lemon
2 tablespoons chopped parsley
1 large garlic clove, peeled and sliced
3 tablespoons olive oil
1 pinch chili flakes
Olive oil spray
½ cup cooked brown rice
3 tablespoons pistou (see pistou recipe, page 256)
Lemon wedges, to serve

Combine sardines, lemon zest, 1 tablespoon chopped parsley, sliced garlic, the olive oil, chili flakes, pinch of salt, and 4 grinds black pepper. Marinate in the fridge at least 30 minutes, or up to overnight.

Take the sardines out of the fridge 20 minutes before you want to cook them. Heat grill pan over medium heat and coat with a bit of olive oil spray to make sure the sardines won't stick. Grill sardines for 3 minutes on each side, until very deeply browned and the flesh is just cooked through.

Serve over warm brown rice and garnish with the remaining tablespoon parsley, the pistou, and lemon wedges.

Pan-Seared Sardines with Capers and Lemon

2 tablespoons olive oil
3 fresh sardines, filleted
Salt and pepper
2 tablespoons capers
1 lemon, cut into thin slices

Heat olive oil in a large sauté pan over medium-high heat, and season sardines with salt and pepper.

When the oil is hot but not smoking, add sardines skin-side down, cook 3 minutes, then flip and cook for another minute.

Remove the sardines to a serving plate and add capers and lemon slices to the sauté pan.

Cook the lemon and capers for 3 minutes over high heat, until the capers become crispy and the lemon slices soften.

Pour the caper/lemon sauce over the sardines and enjoy!

Poached Sardines with Lemon and Chili

4 fresh sardines, scaled, gutted, deboned, and filleted
3 garlic cloves, crushed
1 pinch chili flakes
3 strips of lemon zest, removed with a peeler
1 sprig rosemary
Salt
Olive oil (about ½ cup)

Arrange the sardines in the bottom of a small to medium saucepan; they should fit in a single snug layer. Add the next 4 ingredients, a pinch of salt, and enough olive oil to cover the sardines. Turn the heat on medium, bring the oil up to a simmer, then cover, turn off the heat, and let poach until just cooked through. Cooking times will vary depending on the thickness of the sardines, but start checking after 5 minutes.

Clean Bok Choy

3 tablespoons Bragg Liquid Aminos
1 teaspoon finely minced fresh ginger
1 teaspoon finely diced red chili
1 small garlic clove, very finely minced
Juice of ½ lime
6 pieces baby bok choy, rinsed and dried well
1 tablespoon olive oil
Salt and pepper

Combine first five ingredients in a small bowl.

Heat a grill pan over medium-high heat.

Cut the bok choy in half, toss with olive oil, salt, and pepper, and grill until nicely charred and tender, about 5 to 8 minutes.

Turn off the heat, pour over the sauce, and flip the bok choy.

Let sit 3 minutes to cook the sauce a bit before serving.

Roasted Sweet Potato Dessert

1 medium sweet potato
1 tablespoon olive oil
1 tablespoon flax meal

Preheat the oven to 450 degrees.

Place sweet potato directly on the oven's middle rack, and place a foil-lined baking sheet on the rack below to catch any drippings.

Roast for 1 hour.

When cool enough to eat, scoop out the flesh, mix with olive oil and flax meal, and enjoy!

Clean Veggie Chips

. . . .

BEET CHIPS:

2 medium beets

1 sprig rosemary, stem removed and leaves minced

1 tablespoon olive oil

Kosher salt

Preheat the oven to 325 degrees.

Use a mandoline to slice beets as thin as possible.

Toss the beet slices in a bowl with the minced rosemary, olive oil, and a generous pinch of kosher salt.

Arrange the slices in an even layer on two baking sheets, making sure that none of them overlap. If there are leftover slices, use another baking sheet.

Place the baking sheets in the upper and lower third of the oven, bake for 10 minutes, then switch their positions and bake for another 10 minutes.

Let chips cool on the baking sheets before eating.

KALE CHIPS:

1 bunch curly kale, ribs removed

4 teaspoons olive oil

Harissa powder (if you can't find harissa powder, substitute hot
smoked paprika)
Kosher salt

Preheat the oven to 300 degrees.

Wash and dry the kale well, then tear into large pieces.

Divide kale pieces between two large baking sheets and toss each
batch with 2 teaspoons olive oil, a pinch of harissa powder, and a
generous pinch of kosher salt.

Use your fingers to massage the oil and seasoning into the kale
leaves, then spread out in an even layer, making sure that no pieces
overlap.

Place the baking sheets in the lower and upper thirds of the oven,
bake for 10 minutes, then switch the baking sheets and bake for a
further 7 minutes.

Let the chips cool on the baking sheet before eating.

The "Being" List

The highest state of being is when we are empty and whatever we are experiencing can pour easily into us. In this state, great works of art—whether books, poems, movies, music—can change how we think and even who we are. This list includes my recommendations for works you can read, watch, and experience that will help you continue to cultivate clarity and embody that empty state of being.

BOOKS

The Biology of Belief: Unleashing the Power of Consciousness, Matter & Miracles, by Bruce Lipton, PhD

Lipton, a research scientist and former medical school professor, flips conventional thinking on its head when he contends that our biology is not actually controlled by our DNA, but that our DNA is subject to the energetic messages radiating from our thoughts, be they positive or negative. This groundbreaking work examines a wide range of scientific research into the mind-body connection and makes a compelling and convincing case that, by changing our thinking, we can truly change our biology.

The Body Keeps the Score: Brain, Mind, and Body in the Healing of Trauma, by Bessel van der Kolk, MD

Professor of psychiatry and founder of the Trauma Center in Brookline, Massachusetts, Van der Kolk offers a new way of looking at the traumas that every human being endures at some point in their life. His research shows that trauma literally changes us, reshaping the body and rewiring the brain. But that doesn't mean that we are at the mercy of our most difficult life experiences. The author explores, through stories of veterans, victims of physical violence, and others, not just what happens, but innovative new ways of recovering by activating the brain's own natural capacity for neuroplasticity.

The Evolution of Consciousness: The Origins of the Way We Think, by Robert Ornstein

You wouldn't guess it from the title of the book, but this work deeply facilitated my spiritual awakening. In it, Ornstein seeks to solve the mystery of why the human race experienced a sudden and drastic change in brain size and capability during the Stone Age. At one point, brain size jumped from 600–750 cubic centimeters to an astonishing 775–1,225 cubic centimeters. While the answer to Ornstein's question is intriguing, equally so is the idea he poses that this evolutionary leap created a unique problem for the human race. He states that the physical environment that facilitated our accelerated brain growth ceased to exist a long time ago. Instead, our supercharged brains have created a world that our minds and bodies have not had adequate time to adapt to. This makes sense when we look at the state of the world and all the immense problems so-called advancements have created. Luckily the author has his own suggestions.

The Forty Rules of Love: A Novel of Rumi, by Elif Shafak

This novel follows Ella, an unhappy housewife and reader of manuscripts for a literary agency, who is caught in the grind of her daily routine. Through a synchronous series of events, Ella soon finds herself corresponding via email with Aziz Zahara, the author of the latest manuscript she's reading. Ella and Aziz, a freelance Sufi photographer, begin a dialogue that mirrors the author's latest book, *Sweet Blasphemy*. The book is a bit of historical fiction in which Rumi undergoes a profound transformation after meeting the boisterous Shams and learning his Forty Rules of Love. After becoming versed in them, the previously introverted Rumi becomes a rebel mystic and invents the ecstatic dance of the whirling dervishes in addition to writing his world-renowned poetry.

The message behind the story is that spiritual growth often requires breaking out of one's shell and leaving one's comfort zone behind. As

Ella makes her way through the manuscript and her relationship with Aziz grows, she finds herself faced with the same challenge. Ultimately, this book asks the question, "What is the nature of true spiritual love in our relationships with God, friends, lovers, family members, and even things?" Some of the answers might seem obvious, but just when you think you have them all figured out, you are taken in a direction you would never expect.

A General Theory of Love, by Thomas Lewis, Fari Amini, and Richard Lannon

Three psychiatrists come together to prove scientifically that real health and happiness aren't possible without love. Combining neuroscience with human experience, the authors cleverly and conclusively show that what artists, poets, and musicians have been telling us for millennia about love is scientifically valid on a psychological level. This book crystallized love for me in a tangible way and proved that it's far more than just an ethereal concept. That's why I consider it to be what I call "spiritual nutrition." It's essential for good health and even survival.

In a straightforward way, the authors show that the requirements for loving and healing are exactly the same. One of the most important is maintaining a sense of curiosity. When something unexpected happens, we tend to shun the experience because it wasn't part of our plan. Healing and receiving love require staying open to whatever comes and not being saturated with a lot of pre-scripted expectations. By not limiting ourselves to the answer we want, we remain open to the answer we need to arrive. Like love, when we drop all our prerequisites for what it should be and look like, it will arrive for us, too.

Love: What Life Is All About..., by Leo Buscaglia

I was lucky enough to have Leo Buscaglia as one of my teachers along my life path. He and his landmark book taught me many things about love, mainly that it is the social lubricant that can make any situation work. He offers this unique perspective on social psychology and says that experiencing love requires dropping our defenses. When we can become comfortable with vulnerability and inquisitiveness, we become open and able to receive. He recognizes that this innocent openness with which we are born is shut down, discouraged, and stunted for most of us very early in life. Because of this, most of us are left wanting love but not being able to find or recognize it when it comes. But we can learn, Buscaglia assures us, and his book shows us how.

A special emphasis is put on self-love, which I also promote as an essential part of healing. Buscaglia does a great job of showing us how to love ourselves and pointing out that it's precisely our individual oddities that make us lovable. Ultimately, he says that love is open arms, and if you close your arms about you, you'll find you're left holding only yourself. The central point of all the love there is, is you.

Man's Search for Meaning, by Viktor Frankl

Frankl's bestselling memoir about his time in a Nazi concentration camp can serve as motivation for anyone searching to create new meaning in their lives. Frankl was able to do this in the harshest of circumstances for the sake of his own spiritual survival, and his journey has inspired millions since then.

The Moral Molecule: How Trust Works, by Paul J. Zak

This professor of economic psychology came to be known as the "vampire economist" because of his habit of taking blood samples in order to try to answer a question about what drives trust among people in a society. Through his research, Zak determined that there was a master switch for this human behavior—the hormone oxytocin, which makes us more loving, more trusting, more caring, more generous. All in all, it creates what we would generally describe as "moral behavior."

People of the Lie: The Hope for Healing Human Evil and *The Road Less Traveled*, by M. Scott Peck, MD

Psychiatrist and author Peck explores the nature of love, spiritual growth, and even the human capacity for evil in these books. Peck's insight into and compassion for the human condition will help readers gain a higher level of understanding about themselves.

Rumi: Soul Fury—Rumi and Shams Tabriz on Friendship, by Coleman Barks

Personifying the balance of opposites, the introspective, peaceful Rumi maintained a lifelong friendship with his teacher, the brash and wildly honest Shams Tabriz. That's the relationship at the center of this book by Coleman Barks, the foremost authority on the interpretation and translation of the works of 13th-century Persian poet Rumi. Barks titled his book *Soul Fury* after being inspired by Shams' brand of fiery and passionate spirituality.

The book is an essential collection of short poems from both men on the idea of love as a way of life. For them, truly understanding love required an earnest commitment to the practice of mindfulness, as well as experiencing love in its most profound form as soul friendship. Such a union transcends time and space and is clearly indicative of their own friendship. Many people pass through our lives and intimate relationships often come and go, but it is our true friends that provide us with both grounding and the richness of human experience. There is much to be said about the comfort of not needing to explain ourselves to our lifelong friends because we are at home in their presence. They just get us. This book also makes an excellent gift for a friend who makes you feel exactly this way.

FILMS

Caddyshack (1980): This classic has plenty of mood-elevating comedy that can boost your oxytocin levels, alongside a dose of philosophy, particularly in the "be the ball" scene.

Children of Heaven (1997): A beautiful family drama showing how suffering can bring a family closer together.

The Color of Paradise (1999): This Iranian drama centers on a blind boy whose greatest wish in life is to see God.

Field of Dreams (1989): "If you build it, they will come" is the central message of this classic drama, which is just the way I think about building one's emotional waste management system: if you build it, clarity will come.

Human (2015): Filmmaker Yann Arthus-Bertrand spent several years traveling the world to gather real-life stories that would help answer the question, "What makes us human?" The result is a collection of films that are uplifting, heartbreaking, and always poignant. A convicted murderer's story of "love from the mostly unlikely place" (which can be viewed on the filmmaker's YouTube channel) is a lesson in forgiveness that you won't soon forget.

The Intouchables (2011): It's worth watching this French film for the dancing scene alone, which is practically guaranteed to raise your oxytocin level. I measured, and mine went up four points.

My Dinner with Andre (1981): Part comedy, part drama, this film directed by Louis Malle takes place at a restaurant in New York, where two characters meet for dinner and engage in a ranging conversation that covers the theater, their different personal experiences, and the meaning of life.

Taste of Cherry (1997): This award-winning film centers on a suicidal man scouring the city of Tehran to find someone to do a special job for him: bury him after he takes his own life.

Meditation Moments

The following words of wisdom are meant to inspire and motivate you to reflect inward and experience the majestic beauty of love in a state of consciousness that we've come to know as clarity.

"All great and beautiful work has come from first gazing without shrinking into the darkness."

—John Ruskin, art critic and painter

"Fixing yourself is a task you will never complete because your quest is founded on a faulty premise. You cannot fix yourself because you are not broken."   *—Alan Cohen, author*

"Love dissolves negativity by re-contextualizing it rather than attacking it. This is true happiness."

—David Hawkins, MD, PhD

"For behind all seen things lies something vaster. Everything is but a path, a portal, or a window opening on something more than itself."   *—Antoine de Saint-Exupéry, French writer*

"Freedom is not worth having if it does not include the freedom to err."   *—Mahatma Gandhi*

"There is nothing either good or bad, but thinking makes it so."
—*William Shakespeare,* Hamlet

"It's not what happens to you but how you react to it that matters."
—*Epictetus, Greek philosopher*

"Destiny is no matter of chance, it's a matter of choice."
—*William Jennings Bryan, American politician*

"Live today. Not yesterday. Not tomorrow. Just today. Inhabit your moments. Don't rent them out to tomorrow."
—*Jerry Spinelli, children's author*

"It's not how much we give, but how much love we put into giving."
—*Mother Teresa*

"It's never too late to become what you might have been."
—*George Eliot, novelist*

"Adopt the pace of nature: her secret is patience."
—*Ralph Waldo Emerson*

"I will love the light, for it shows me the way. Yet, I will endure the darkness for it shows me the stars."
—*Og Mandino, author*

"The spirit is the master; imagination the tool, and the body the plastic material...The power of the imagination is a great factor in medicine. It may produce diseases in man and in animals, and it may cure them. Ills of the body may be cured by physical remedies or by the power of the spirit acting through the soul."—*Paracelsus*

Acknowledgments

i gathered in a fluttering throng on a cancerous dark night,

To consider gaining some clarity around a candle light.

There were mentors, many, who appeared to guide me
which way to go,
To gather some news of the elusive Healing glow.

(My Beloved Parents: Manijeh & Gholamhossein, Dr. H. Mehran Sadeghi, Dr. H. Mehrdad Sadeghi, Dr. Gary Rueles, Mr. Mehdi Sarreshtehdari, Dr. Jean Claude Lapraz, Mr. Kamran Golestaneh, Mrs. Annette Davis, Mr. Raha Hasti, Mr. Eric Davis, Mr. & Mrs. Emami, Dr. Stefan Hagopian, Mr. Luke Cowles, Dr. John Sharifi, Mr. Hutch Morton, Mr. Coleman Barks, Ms. Lisa Starr)

As i flew, in the distance, i discerned,
A palace window where a clear candle burned.
And went no nearer: back again,
i enthusiastically flew,
To wanna tell others what i thought
i knew.

There were even more mentors, appearing then,
substantiating my claim,
honoring that: "yes, yes, he has seen the flame."

(Mr. Werner Erhard, Mr. Yehuda Naftali, Mrs. Byron Katie Mitchell, Dr. Gary David, Mr. David Booth, Mrs. Deborah Shames, Dr. Christian Duraffourd, Dr. Kamyar Hedayat, Drs. Ron and Mary Hulnick, my beloved masterful teachers, who have helped me immensely to give birth to much of the linguistic abstraction of *The Clarity Cleanse* (and grateful for our healing intentional community at USM). Mrs. Johanna Jenkins, Dr. Jon Tabakin, Mr. Sidi M. al-Jamal, Dr. Morton Herskowitz, Mr. Stevollah F. Hardison, Dr. Habib Davanloo, Mrs. Celeste Fine, Mr. John Maas, Dr. John Davies, Mrs. Christa Bourg, Mr. David Robert Ord, Ms. Karen Murgolo, and Hachette Book Group)

A more eager me than the one before,
Set out and passed beyond the palace door.

As i hovered in the clear aura of that fire,
A trembling blur of timorous desire,
Then rapidly headed back to let others know, how far i had been,
And how much clarity, i had seen.

(Ms. Gwyneth Paltrow and goop family, Mr. Christopher A. J. Martin)

Then there was another me who flew out on a dizzy flight,
Turned to an ardent wooing of the clear light;

As that me dipped and soared,
Both self and fire mingled.

As the flame engulfed my body and head,
My being tingled a fierce translucent red;

Here, sat, few mentors who saw my sudden blaze,
And witnessed my mindset, shifting, Clearer, within glowing rays.

"He knows, he knows, the clarity we all seek,
That which is hidden and no one can speak."

(Mr. Shervine Dowlatshahi, Mrs. Vivian Liu, MegaZEN Team, Love Button Global Movement Family, Be Hive of Healing Family including every single patient I have had the privilege of serving since 1995, And Last and Most: My Sweet Beloveds, Dr. Shahrzad (Sherry) Sami Dowlatshahi, Hafez & HannaH Sami-Sadeghi)

Forever indebted, I Am, to The Light of Light and all of my mentors who pushed me beyond all knowledge to find,
The Clarity Cleanse, that Love that once eluded my mind.
Dr. Habib Sadeghi (with help from mystic poet Attar.)
Father's Day
2017

About the Author

Dr. Habib Sadeghi
Fellow of the American Society of Endobiogenic
Medicine and Integrative Physiology

HABIB SADEGHI, DO, FACEMIP, is the cofounder of Be Hive of Healing, an integrative medical health center in Agoura Hills, and the Love Button Global Movement. With a Masters in Spiritual Psychology with Emphasis in Consciousness, Health, and Healing from the University of Santa Monica, he provides a comprehensive knowledge of revolutionary healing protocols in integrative, osteopathic, anthroposophical, environmental, psychosomatic, and family medicine. Through a unique and individualized approach to health care, Dr. Sadeghi has been able to achieve astounding results in patient cases that were otherwise deemed hopeless. His success in integrating Eastern and Western healing practices has earned him a respected reputation resulting in a patient base that reaches around the world.

Dr. Sadeghi served as an attending physician at UCLA Medical Center, Santa Monica, and is currently a clinical instructor of family medicine at Western University of Health Sciences. Having personally experienced miraculous results from the use of integrative medicine, he passionately promotes these protocols among residents and medical students. He is a member of the Physicians' Association for Anthroposophic Medicine and International Postgraduate Medical Training for Anthroposophic Medicine. An active member of the Price-Pottenger Nutrition Foundation and American Holistic Medical Association, he is regularly sought after as an expert in the fields of psychosomatic medicine, nutritional therapy, dietary supplementation, and detoxification for chronic conditions such as heart disease, cancer, and autoimmune diseases.

Dr. Sadeghi has conducted health and wellness conferences throughout the US, Canada, and Europe that draw capacity crowds. He is also one of the first osteopathic physicians to be invited to present at the internationally televised fundraiser Stand Up to Cancer (SU2C). He is the author of *Within: A Spiritual Awakening to Love & Weight Loss* and *Seeds of the Soul: Inspirations for a Life in Healing Transition.* He is also a contributor to the book *The Light,* along with Don Miguel Ruiz, Terry Tillman, Barbara Marx Hubbard, John-Roger, and other leaders in health and spirituality. He is a regular contributor to goop and the Huffington Post and serves as the publisher of *MegaZEN,* an annual health and wellness journal.

For more information, go to BeingClarity.com.